Changing Human Behavior

Strategies
for Preventive
Dentistry

Philip Weinstein, Ph.D.
Assistant Professor, Department of Community Dentistry
University of Washington School of Dentistry
Seattle, Washington

Tracy Getz, M.S.
Lecturer, Department of Community Dentistry
University of Washington School of Dentistry
Seattle, Washington

The C. V. Mosby Company

ST. LOUIS • TORONTO • LONDON   1978

Copyright © 1978 by The C. V. Mosby Company

All rights reserved. No part of this book may be reproduced
in any manner without written permission of the publisher.

Printed in the United States of America

The C. V. Mosby Company
11830 Westline Industrial Drive, St. Louis, Missouri 63141

Library of Congress Catalog Number   78-57597
ISBN 0-8016-5405-X

Cover and Text Design by James A. Buddenbaum
Illustrations by Robert Keys

CB/CB   9   8   7   6   5   4   3   2   1   01/D/095

Contents

Lots of folks confuse bad management with destiny.
 E. Hubbard

Preface

It sometimes seems that there is an endless parade of articles, books, and continuing education courses about how to motivate patients. Such presentations exhort us to use this or that approach to educate patients and convince them that they should change what they are doing in order to achieve better dental health. These presentations are exciting and stimulate us to try harder at developing better plaque control and other programs, and if you are like many readers of this book you have already tried more than one approach to such preventive dentistry. And as each approach fails, we hesitate, and decide to try one more time. We buy expensive visual aids, pamphlets, and even phase-contrast microscopes. We spend time with patients demonstrating proper techniques and talking about the importance of brushing, flossing, and having adequate nutrition. Initially, patients seem to respond. They nod their heads in agreement, and think "it is a good idea" too. Some patients actually attempt to follow our new programs. At last, a successful preventive practice!

However, a week or perhaps even a month later the approach seems to fail. We find that although many patients are reluctant to admit it, they have been unable to carry through the program over a prolonged period of time. Frustrated again! Isn't there anything that works? If you spend some time talking to your colleagues you may find that many of them have given up worrying about prevention. But, since you have read this far, it may be safe to assume that you are still searching for a successful approach.

This book was written to help dental health care providers and students. The techniques and principles presented in the following pages can be applied by any member of a dental health team. However, as with any procedure, the entire staff must support the prevention program. Because of the very nature of their jobs, auxiliaries have considerable contact time with patients and sometimes find it easier than the dentist to apply procedures like the ones discussed in this book.

Each office is run differently. In some, the dentist and auxiliaries share equally in work with prevention; in others, prevention is assigned almost exclusively to the auxiliary staff. A word of caution: As patients usually assign 'ultimate authority' to the dentists, it is important that dentists make clear their support for the prevention program and that patients realize the prevention program is a vital part of the overall treatment plan.

In the last two decades, much research has been conducted on how and why people change their behavior and habits. The principles and techniques discovered have been successfully applied in a variety of educational, psychological, and medical settings. In this book we apply these principles to the field of dentistry.*

To help patients change their poor dental self-care, it is not enough merely to help them think in different ways or even to 'motivate' them to try something new. Doing something just once to prevent future problems is not too difficult. Most of us, for example, are willing to be inoculated to prevent contracting an infectious disease during an epidemic. However, most of us also find it very difficult to start and keep doing some new, extra task regularly, or to stop a habit or something we enjoy in order to reduce the chances of some future problem. Though new knowledge may change our thinking, and professionals and others may provide some initial encouragement, we are unable to make a sustained effort over what seems an infinite period of time. How many of us have made unsuccessful New Year's resolutions to stop smoking, or broken one diet after another, or started an aerobic exercise program only to quit a week or two later? It's not hard for any of us to identify what we should or should not do, or even to try to change. But it is extremely difficult to build a preventive habit that lasts.

* The authors are greatly indebted to such psychologists, as Bandura, Premack, and Skinner, who identified basic principles of human behavior, and to those psychologists who successfully applied these principles to a variety of important human problems, e.g., Becker, Bijou, Ferster, Homme, Lindsley, Mager, and Patterson.

This book is designed to help you and your patients establish lasting preventive habits and eliminate dysfunctional or harmful habits. Our approach is practical, not theoretical. We are not presenting an approach that will immediately replace your existing plaque control or preventive program. We are presenting a system that suggests a wide range of techniques which we believe you will find useful with particular patients. We ask you not to accept our entire approach uncritically. The techniques and basic principles used are illustrated with numerous examples. However, just as reading a book about fly fishing will not put trout in your creel, simply reading this book is not enough.

We believe you can best learn and understand our approach and techniques by trying them out. Consequently, we will ask you to identify a real problem you want to work on as you read this book. By following the principles and techniques presented, you will be able to successfully design and implement a program to manage the problem you have identified, and learn how to apply the same techniques and principles to other human problems. From there, it should be possible to help your patients manage their problems, with a view to improving their dental health.

P.W. & T.G.

I want to change things.
I want to see them happen.
I don't want just to talk about them.
  J. K. Galbraith

Introduction

The Basic Issues
and the Basic Steps

Issue I Is Preventive
Dentistry Possible

As a health professional, you spend much of your time trying to change your patients' old habits and to help them establish new ones. Although they may want to do so, many patients do not floss or even brush regularly. Caries-susceptible children and young adults often are not able to stop eating tasty cariogenic snacks. Adults frequently are not able to stop or even decrease smoking. Older children are often unable to cease their thumbsucking or other harmful oral habits.

Even when compliance is easily within their power, patients do not always comply with professional recommendations. For example: A surprising number of patients may not do something so simple as ingesting a small tablet or applying an ointment once a day with regularity. With more difficult tasks, such as the changing of eating habits or the cessation of smoking, the number of noncomplying patients is staggering. In addition, patients often do not show up for regular dental care. Some are extremely fearful; a large number are just anxious.

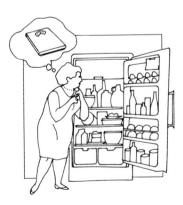

Patients' late arrivals, cancellations, broken appointments, and similar problems are frustrating for both practitioners and students.

After an extensive review of the research literature, Drs. Sackett and Haynes reported in 1976 that 30% to 70% of all recommendations for medication, diet, exercise, and/or home care are *not* followed by patients. There is no question that noncompliance is a serious problem, for the two major diseases of the oral cavity, periodontitis and caries, are controllable—and possibly preventable—with the active cooperation of the patients. A pioneer in the study of patient compliance, Dr. Milton Davis, reported in 1966 that when practitioners are questioned about the compliance of their own patients, they grossly underestimate the extent of the problem and they do not acknowledge—or don't know—that many of their own recommendations are ignored.

The problem boils down to this: Patients, though they may want to, are not behaving the way you, and in many cases they, know they should. It seems that at one point or another all people do not comply with professional advice. As Pogo, the sage of the comic strip, once noted, "We have met the enemy, and they is us."

As practitioners, our solutions for this basic problem are often not satisfactory. Using our authority to direct a patient to maintain some level of home care and clinic attendance, or to seek care elsewhere, may temporarily relieve our frustration, but it does little to solve the patient's problem. Similarly, we may find that educational and motivational approaches in which patients are given information and encouragement can result in new patient insight but, all too often, elicit little lasting change. A patient's desire to cooperate may not be enough to effect lasting change. It is apparent that new techniques are needed to deal with these problems.

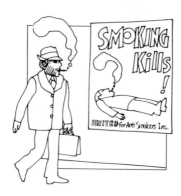

In this book, we present systematic procedures for changing behavior—procedures based on the results of hundreds of research studies conducted in many different health care settings. We offer ways to understand and apply the techniques of **behavior management** or modification—procedures used by an ever-increasing number of health professionals and lay people whose concern is why people behave as they do and how behavior can be positively changed in order to promote good health. Because this book emphasizes the practical application of skills, we offer you opportunities for practice before you apply the skills to patient care. We do this by suggesting a project in which you identify a real problem and then design and implement a program to manage and change it by using certain techniques. We believe that talking about how to handle problems, or even watching others solve them, though useful, is not enough. Just as having someone describe a clinic or laboratory procedure, or even present a film or videotape describing it, is not a substitute for the 'hands on' experience of doing the procedure yourself.

In summary, as preventive dentistry requires long-standing change in human behavior, inherent difficulties should be expected. Nonetheless, there are techniques which can be used to enhance the overall success of a preventive program. Using these techniques in the dental setting is what this book is all about.

Issue II Is It Ethical to Change Patient Behavior

Since this book focuses on the acquisition of skills that can be used in changing behavior, you may be concerned about the ethics of manipulating other people's behavior.

Practitioners often ask, "Do I have a right to intervene or try to persuade a patient to work on a problem? Does my responsibility stop at identifying and informing a patient about a problem?" What about motivation? Some health professionals feel that if their patients "really wanted to do it" or had "enough motivation" or "willpower" they could change, and that the professional's intervention would be unnecessary.

It is our position that if the dental health professional can help a patient to recognize a problem, and if the patient expresses a desire to change, the health professional should facilitate the patient's attempt at changing his behavior through the use of specific techniques. To phrase it another way: Once the patient expresses the desire to change, the practitioner can supply some expertise in *how* to effect that change.

In working with another person to help him change old habits or establish new behavior, we are not working against the individual's will. In fact, we are doing just the opposite: working with an individual to help him accomplish what he realizes is in his best interest. Moreover, helping an individual to break old habits or establish new ones strengthens the person's confidence in his ability to control his own life. We are the means by which a patient can meet his desired ends. The techniques that we will present are part of a systematic six-step approach that can help people to reach acceptable, ethical objectives and develop their abilities to change themselves.

Finally, it is important to reiterate that behavior change programs seldom can work effectively without the active cooperation of the person for whom the change is desired. If the person does not acknowledge ownership of a problem, or if there is not an objective that he desires or believes is worth working towards, a behavior change program will have little chance of success.

Motivating the Patient

Motivation is a term which means many different things to many people. When we speak of motivating patients, the term connotes external influence or inducement to change. Usually we think of dental health care providers attempting to.motivate patients to think and act in ways that may ultimately result in their performing a preventive behavior habitually. We see this as an ethical end. What are the means? The act of motivating a patient involves generating interest, showing your concern, and providing information.

Many ways exist to generate interest. Audiovisual materials, phase-contrast microscopes, and other instruments are useful; however, our own interest in prevention is probably the most important factor. If we are not enthusiastic about what we are doing, we communicate this attitude to the patient. Similarly, concern about the welfare of the patient is important. Patients usually judge concern by the amount of time the health professional spends talking to them about their health and their problems. The information provided need not be technical, but it must be relevant. Patients need to understand why we see the information as important and how it relates to them personally. In short, to maximize the chances of motivating the patient to think and act in different ways, the message must be personalized, not 'canned'.

Behavior Change

Patient motivation	Change in	Initiation of	Behavior
Health professional's →	patient's →	patient's new →	becomes
interest	thoughts	behavior	a habit
concern			
information			

This chart illustrates the entire process of change. First, we motivate patients to change their thoughts and to act—that is, to try out the new **behaviors** in flossing, brushing, and diet. After the patients act, we attempt to make the new behavior part of their regular daily routine—a **habit.**

As we continue our discussion of the ethics of motivation, it might be useful to view the issue from the perspective of problem **ownership.** Whose problem is it? Does the patient feel that his lack of home care is a problem for him? Or are you, the health professional, the only one who is aware of the problem and concerned about the patient's home care? Will a change meet the needs recognized and desired by the patient, or only your objectives as a health professional? It is critical that the health professional always examine the ownership of any given problem. Once a patient owns a problem—or sees a behavior as a problem with consequences for himself—he will take responsibility for, and will attempt to follow advice about solving, the problem. When a patient has no sense of ownership or concern about consequences, most attempts to motivate him fail and lead to frustration.

If the state of the patient's oral health bothers you but not the patient, there are some strategies that are more effective than others, and less intrusive on the patient's integrity. At first, do not attempt to educate, motivate, or otherwise persuade such patients of the legitimacy of your recommendations. Criticizing, blaming, or disagreeing with the patient will not help either. Remember, this patient feels he is doing what is best for him—he feels no need to change. Instead, it may be best to talk to the patient about your problem and your concerns. Instead of telling the patient, "You should or should not . . .", or "You are not taking good care of your teeth", it would be more effective to eliminate 'you-messages' as well as the editorial 'we' and substitute 'I-messages'. For example: "I would like you to . . .", or "It bothers me . . .", or "I enjoy working with patients who take care of their teeth", or "I get discouraged when I see you don't brush regularly." Such statements of your feelings are apt to provoke less resistance. To communicate the effect of the patient's behavior on you is far less threatening than to suggest that there is something unacceptable about what the patient is doing. Moreover, the patient now has the responsibility to respond to *your* feelings. As a result of this mild face-to-face confrontation, negotiation becomes possible.

If the patient does not respond, it may be best not to press the attempt to change his behavior. On a given day, you cannot expect every one of your patients to desire to change their oral habits. Such unrealistic expectations inevitably lead to frustration which paradoxically lessens wholehearted commitments to your preventive program. Many people, especially those who are under some form of stress, are not prepared to undertake change or to disturb their present routine. Perhaps at some time in the future, their life circumstances will have changed and they will be ready.

Once patients own the problem, another ownership question is this: How much responsibility should dental health professionals take to help the patients change their behavior? If a patient attempts to change and fails, is it the professional's fault? Determination of ownership is critical. The practitioner cannot succeed if the patient does not verbally acknowledge a need to deal with the problem. (Passive patient acquiescence often leads to future problems.) However, when patients do own the problem, we believe health professionals are responsible to do everything within their power to facilitate a successful change program for their patients. Health professionals cannot be responsible for the behavior of the patient when he has no desire to change. Instead, their responsibility is to work with the patient who desires change.

When the patient owns only part of the problem, how hard should the practitioner work at motivating a patient —convincing or persuading him of the problem and the need to change his behavior? This is a question which can be answered only by each individual practitioner. However, the more the push for change comes from the practitioner, and not the patient, the less likely is success.

Once the patient has fully acknowledged ownership of a problem, and the health professional has helped motivate him to change his behavior, a plan for changing the behavior can be formulated.

The Basic Steps of Behavior Change

When we speak of **behavior,** we are talking about actions. Behavior that is repeated regularly and has become part of one's daily routine is what we know in everyday life as habit. In the following situations, the regularly repeated behaviors are **habits** people would like to change, but . . . .

"Diane, I've *got* to quit smoking. I'm just getting too short of breath to get up these stairs, and I know that smoking's not good for me. I'm going to stop, starting today."
   "Great! Maybe you'll really stop this time."
   "I'll start Monday, after your party."

"Jack doesn't show me as much attention as he used to. He always has an excuse. If I only could lose a little weight, about 20 pounds. Maybe if I starved myself for a week. Some people get their jaws wired shut to stop them from eating—I wonder if my dentist. . . . "

"Oh, honey, I can't exercise with you today. I've got too much work to do, and I have to go to the office."

"Oh, George, not again. You promised. Remember? You said you would run with me every day, and this is the third day in a row that you haven't. Doesn't it bother you to look the way you do? You'll never lose any weight. I hate going all alone."

"O.K., we're done for now, Mr. Farnsworth. But remember, you've *got* to start brushing and flossing regularly, or you're going to have very serious problems with your teeth."

Do these situations sound familiar? People often do have real problems in changing their own behavior and the behavior of others. Stop for a few moments to do a quick exercise.

Try to list recent examples where you tried to change your own behavior, or that of your friends or relatives.

What behavior have you tried to change in your patients?

What kinds of problems have you faced while trying to change behavior in yourself or others?

As a health professional, you are intimately involved with patient dental care habits, and you are continually in the position of attempting to modify the care patients give to their mouths.

How to Do This — The Six Fundamental Steps.

In seeking any change, we increase our chance of success by approaching the change process systematically. We have divided the process of changing behavior into six fundamental steps that provide just such an orderly system.

1. Identifying and specifically defining the problem. Determining the nature of the problem is essential. Does it involve a lack of knowledge? A lack of skills? For example, Ms. Fields has periodontal problems and an accumulation of calculus and plaque on her teeth. You would determine whether: she has the skill to brush properly; she recognizes the importance of home care; and she feels the need to take better care of her teeth.

2. Planning to collect baseline data. Before attempting to initiate any change, it is important to find out specific instances of when and where the behavior occurs, or does not occur. For example, Ms. Fields, who has the needed skills and desire, may not be aware that she almost never brushes her teeth on weekends and when she is rushed in the mornings.

3. Specifying goals and objectives. In this step we determine and set specific realistic objectives that can be reached. Instead of requesting Ms. Fields to brush and floss more often or better, it is more effective to specify a definite and realistic number of times per week. For example, Ms. Fields, who brushes twice a week, may be successful in increasing her brushings to four times a week. Requesting her to start brushing and flossing every day may be too high a goal to strive for initially and would only result in feelings of failure. In working with a patient you develop short as well as long-range objectives. For Ms. Fields, brushing daily may be a realistic long-range objective for her to work towards. Increasing her brushings to four times a week might be an initial and, from her point of view, achievable intermediate objective.

4. Planning an intervention. In this stage you decide what you will actually do to help change the pinpointed behavior. In the case of Ms. Fields, this could involve any number of strategies, such as: setting up cues to brush, changing the time and place of the brushing habit, and having her provide herself with rewards for brushing that are strong enough to influence her to act. These strategies and others are fully discussed in chapter 4.

5. Monitoring and modifying the plan. One should not assume that the intervention will work flawlessly. Monitoring or gathering data about the rate of progress is extremely helpful. For example, when recording and charting her brushing, Ms. Fields may find that her intervention is not having the full effect desired. After investigating or troubleshooting the problem, she may modify the intervention or alter intermediate objectives to reflect what may realistically be accomplished.

6. Planning for termination. In this phase of the formal change project, arrangements are made for the patient's self-maintenance of the new behavior. The end must be as carefully planned as the beginning to help the patient avoid backsliding.

Although these six fundamental steps appear to be distinct from one another, they are in fact closely related. We have placed the six steps in a framework that permits you to accomplish your role in them during part of four contact sessions with the patient, noting the session in which each step can be accomplished.

As Part of the Step

1st Session	1. Identifying and specifically defining the problem
	2. Planning to collect baseline data
2nd Session	3. Specifying goals and objectives
	4. Planning an intervention
3rd Session	5. Monitoring and modifying the plan
4th Session	6. Planning for termination

For clarification and for quick reference when you are actually designing projects for your practice, a summary of the steps and sessions is presented in Appendix A.

You have probably noticed that in the six steps discussed above there is no mention of communication skills or of establishing rapport. These interpersonal relation skills are important; in fact, none of the procedures in this book can be successfully applied without them. Although, we have purposely omitted these topics, nonetheless the bibliography includes references on communication skills in the dental setting if you are interested in further information in this area.

In summary, long-term preventive programs can be implemented for patients who desire to change. For those who for whatever reason are not amenable to change, pressing the issue will result in failure and frustration. Helping patients who desire to change is ethical, and the means are within the realm of the dental professional. The six fundamental steps by which lasting change may be accomplished have been outlined and will be discussed in detail in the six following chapters.

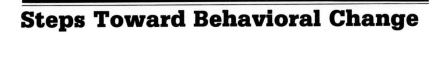

Steps Toward Behavioral Change

It isn't that they can't see the solution.
It is that they can't see the problem.
  G. K. Chesterton

1 The First Step

Identifying and Specifically Defining the Problem

In session one, the practitioner can identify and define the problem.

Performance Discrepancies

If we stop and look around us, one conclusion is inescapable. Life is filled with many discrepancies. There are discrepancies between what we are told and what we know to be true, between our desires and our abilities, between what we intend to do and what we actually do. A gap between desired performance and actual performance is called a **performance discrepancy.*** When we identify and choose a problem to work on, it will usually involve such a discrepancy. If so, then we must further define the discrepancy.

When we find a patient who is not flossing, wearing headgear, or using an appliance, we often assume that he either does not know how to do it, or he does not know how important it is, for if he did, he would obviously be doing it! After all, it is for his own benefit. For example, instructors are often heard saying, "We've got to motivate our students to turn in their work on time." Pedodontists have

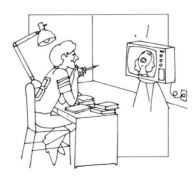

* The authors gratefully acknowledge the work of Robert Mager, who coined this term and popularized the problem solving approach that is the basis of this chapter.

been heard saying to their assistants, "We've got to teach parents that sugar snacks aren't good for their children's teeth." Prosthodontists have been heard to say to orthodontists, "We've got to motivate our patients to wear their appliances consistently." And oral pathologists have been overheard talking to themselves, "We've got to teach the public that smoking is harmful."

Students know they are supposed to turn in their work on time; parents know certain snacks may cause cavities; patients know they should wear their appliances; and all of us know the relationship between smoking and cancer.

Approaches to performance discrepancies that are based upon statements such as, "We've got to teach, educate, or motivate," are usually unproductive. Such statements talk about solutions, not problems. Training, teaching, and instruction in health education are solutions or remedies, for a lack of information. *Frequently, however, lack of information is not the problem.*

Thus, after we identify a performance discrepancy and begin to define it, we must also determine the cause of the discrepancy. This is a critical concern because our interpretation determines the kind of solution we will propose.

Skill Deficiencies vs. Management Deficiencies

The most basic differentiation to make is whether the problem results from a **skill deficiency** or from a **management deficiency.** In other words, why is the patient not performing the desired behavior? To determine this, Mager (1970) suggests we ask two questions: (1) Could the patient perform the desired behavior, e.g., brushing or flossing, if he really had to? (2) Could he do it if his life depended on it? If the answer is "No," for example, the patient cannot demonstrate that he can remove all the stain produced by the disclosing tablet, then there is a genuine skill deficiency for which education or some form of instruction is a critical step—for example, teaching a patient how to brush or floss under his bridge. However, if the answer to the question "Could he do it if he had to?" is "Yes," we then know the patient has the necessary knowledge or skills, and the problem is a management deficiency. Another clue that a problem is a management deficiency rather than a skill deficiency is when we hear ourselves or others saying such things as "He just isn't motivated enough"; "He doesn't seem to really want to do it"; "He doesn't really care"; or "He doesn't have the right attitude." In other words, he is managing his behavior poorly. When the problem is a management deficiency rather than one involving the patient's skills or knowledge, we have to attempt to alter the conditions associated

Steps Toward Behavioral Change

with the performance or the consequences of that performance.

Unfortunately, saying to ourselves or others "You *oughta wanna* do it for your own good" is not a strong motivator for influencing anyone to do anything he already knows how to do, as every cigarette smoker or overweight person can tell us.

It should be pointed out that many of the changes that we as health professionals are concerned with are preventive habits. These preventive habits are especially difficult to establish and maintain. The knowledge that one may avoid a problem in the future is often not a very powerful way to influence what most people do in the present. For example, do you wear a seat belt every time you drive?

Take a minute and look back on those problems you identified in the Introduction. Were they a result of a skill deficiency, a management deficiency, or some combination of the two? Clearly, the course of action will differ for each. If you have identified a patient's problem as a skill deficiency, you are ready to plan an instructional program that will enable the patient to learn the missing skill. That is at least a partial beginning. If you later find that your patient is in fact using the skill, positive behavior change has occurred and you can be pleased that the process was relatively simple.

However, if you find that the skill deficiency has been remediated but the patient is not habitually using the newly learned skill, for example, he does not brush often or does so only superficially, you now have identified a management deficiency which may relate to the quantity (frequency) or quality (adequacy) of home care. It is time to move to step two, to pinpoint the deficiency and collect baseline data about it. (In chapter 4, step four, where we discuss planning and implementing an intervention, there will be some specific procedures to use for developing both new skills and habits.)

Your Practice Project

First Assignment

As we noted in the Preface, we suggest that you identify and work on a change project as you progress through this book. It is always legitimate to ask what kinds of projects are appropriate. The principles of 'behavior change' that are discussed in this book can be used in any setting and with a wide variety of problems.

The intent of this book is not to teach you to be a behavior therapist, nor is that the role or function of the dental health professional. The end result of the methods and techniques discussed in this book is that your patients are helped to practice better home care and you are helped in your management of problematic patient behavior in the health care setting. Thus, our focus is specific identifiable habits and behavior revolving around oral health care and in-office behavior.

Is this talk of 'behavior' and 'habits' superficial? What about personality and the reasons why people do things? This topic has been the center of many debates. As you probably know, having insight, or knowing why we are the way we are or knowing what we should do, rarely leads to significant change. It has been our experience that almost all the problems that concern dental health practitioners involve habits, or the lack of them. Why a particular habit such as smoking or frequent sugar snacking occurs seldom has much relevance to the control of such habits. There are, of course, times when even the simplest behavior seems so complexly linked to what appears to be an overwhelming series of problems that making changes seems too difficult. Some good examples include the patient who is extremely fearful of dental treatment or the patient who is a compulsive eater. Soon after you initiate a project it may become apparent that the problem is too big to handle. In such cases referral to an appropriate therapist is the best course to follow.

Look back on some of the principles of behavior change and use the space on the next page to identify and discuss in writing three problems you, your patients, or your acquaintances are probably willing to own. Remember, you need not try to manufacture hypothetical problems—we all have real problems and know people with real problems worth working on. Some examples of projects with which other practitioners have had success include:

increasing brushing and/or flossing
ceasing or reducing smoking or alcohol consumption
increasing headgear compliance
losing weight
making diet and nutritional changes, especially reduction of cariogenic food
    intake
beginning and carrying out regular exercise programs, such as the aerobics
    program recommended by Cooper (1970)
stopping nailbiting or thumbsucking
increasing study time
decreasing patient anxiety to manageable levels
increasing wearing of dentures
decreasing child misbehavior in the operatory

Assignment I

I. 1. Whose problem is it (patient, spouse, friend, self)?

   2. Describe the problem.
     a. Specify what the person is doing or not doing that needs changing.
     b. Specify the situation (at home, work, clinic; morning, afternoon).

   3. Describe why you believe the problem is a management deficiency.

II. 1. Whose problem is it (patient, spouse, friend, self)?

   2. Describe the problem.
     a. Specify what the person is doing or not doing that needs changing.
     b. Specify the situation (at home, work, clinic; morning, afternoon).

   3. Describe why you believe the problem is a management deficiency.

III. 1. Whose problem is it (patient, spouse, friend, self)?

   2. Describe the problem.
     a. Specify what the person is doing or not doing that needs changing.
     b. Specify the situation (at home, work, clinic; morning, afternoon).

   3. Describe why you believe the problem is a management deficiency.

Half our mistakes in life arise from feeling where we ought to think, and thinking where we ought to feel.
  J. Collins

Many people fail because they conclude that fundamentals do not apply in their case.
  M. L. Cichon

2 The Second Step

Planning to Collect Baseline Data

In session one, the practitioner arranges to have baseline data collected.

The Value of Baseline Counting

What are **baseline counts?** They are counts of behavior taken before a change is initiated. The most important reason for taking a baseline is that the counts enable you to determine later whether or not the change procedure you use is effective.

It might seem to you that any change in behavior would be readily apparent—that there is really no need for an objective verification that comes from taking before-and-after counts. However, often this is not the case. For example, consider the case of the individual in this illustration.

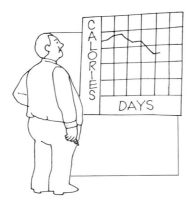

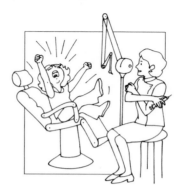

We see that originally the person was consuming approximately 3,500 calories of food per day. In a period of approximately two weeks, after the behavior change project was initiated, the caloric intake decreased to approximately 3,100 calories per day. Although change has occurred and a pattern has been established, it probably would not be observable to the naked eye. Unless baseline data were taken, the person might have become prematurely discouraged and discontinued any efforts to change at all.

Another helpful aspect of baseline data is that they often affect our thinking about the importance of changing a behavior. Sometimes, for example, it may seem as if a patient exhibits disruptive or annoying behavior all the time, or that a child never brushes his teeth. But it is often easy to overreact to certain behavior and to overestimate its frequency. Taking a baseline helps you to determine objectively the seriousness of the problem. In turn, this helps you decide whether or not you want to invest the time and effort involved in initiating a change program.

Sometimes collecting baselines results in a decision not to change a particular behavior, but to leave it alone. For example, you may find that a young patient is not misbehaving as grossly as he seemed to be—he only misbehaves towards the beginning of the appointment (for example, during injections).

Finally, baseline counts will help you to set realistic goals for those you work or live with, or for yourself. When using behavior change procedures, deciding precisely what you want to accomplish in any given situation or how far you want to go is important. For example, for a child who wears headgear only two hours per day when at home, specifying a reachable increment, say three hours per day at home, may be a useful intermediate objective in promoting headgear use. When the child achieves a specified intermediate objective, he feels successful and is likely to attempt further progress. But unless you know how frequently a behavior occurs to start with, it is difficult to set realistic and meaningful objectives for behavior

Steps Toward Behavioral Change

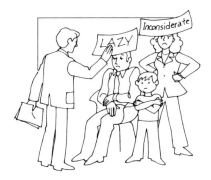

change, and to know objectively when you have achieved your objectives.

Preparing to Count: Pinpointing

Before you begin counting a behavior, you must describe the particular behavior in terms of when and where it occurs or doesn't occur. This is known as **pinpointing,** and it is the first part of taking baseline data. For example, if you are concerned about a patient's seeming lack of home care, and you have determined the problem is not a skill deficiency, you would want to pinpoint when and where the patient does and does not brush and floss.

Pinpointing is important for the very practical reason that behavior change procedures are extremely effective in modifying the course of objective and observable events, events that can be seen or heard. Consequently, it is best to translate your feelings or impressions into pinpointed descriptions of behavior.

If you stray from behavioral observations, it is much too easy to attribute false motivations to others. Patients who do not brush regularly may be seen as lazy, or patients who arrive late for appointments may seem inconsiderate. These labels only get in the way in working with a patient. You must try instead to identify whatever the person is doing or saying which prompts use of these labels. Remember, you are not trying to change someone's personality. You want to change only the behavior that is hampering good dental care. This can be facilitated by keeping in mind several simple questions:

1. What does the individual do or say or fail to do that brings about the problem situation?
2. In what situations, or when and where, does the behavior occur or fail to occur?
3. Is your description of the problem free of words which interpret or explain?
4. Can you count the behavior you described?

Planning to Collect Baseline Data

In every case, your objective is to identify specific behavior you would like to see occur more or less frequently in a particular situation. Take the case of a patient who might be considered lazy or inconsiderate. In the process of pinpointing, you will find that it is what the 'lazy' patient does not do (he does not floss although he knows how to do it) or what the 'inconsiderate' patient does (always arrives ten minutes late for morning appointments) that irritates you. In pinpointing, the situation in which this sort of behavior occurs or does not occur is made clear. It is only then that a plan can be made which will determine how to go about solving the problem.

The final pinpointing question "Can I count or measure the behavior I described?" can help you in two ways. First, a behavior cannot be counted unless it can be seen or heard, so you are helped to focus on behavior. In addition, counting is important because most of our procedures are designed to change the rate of behavior—for example, increasing the number of flossings per week; decreasing the number of between-meal snacks per day; decreasing the number of cigarettes smoked per day; or increasing the number of hours per day of headgear wearing.

Before proceeding, we would like to reiterate a few points made in the Introduction and chapter 1. Determining whether the patient perceives there is a problem and securing agreement to work on the problem is the critical first step that must not be forgotten. If the patient recognizes and owns the problem and verbally agrees with the desirability of change, then it is possible to proceed. If not, or if you are unsure of how the patient views the situation, you should not push ahead.

After dealing with any skill deficits that may exist (see chapter 4), engage the patient in a critical but brief discussion of where and when the behavior in question (usually brushing or flossing) occurs and does not occur. This conversation will set the stage for making arrangements with the patient to collect baseline data—which will pinpoint the problem more explicitly.

Taking the Baseline Count

Basic Considerations. In counting behavior, you should be aware of the fact that it is not always necessary for you to count the behavior in question. There may be times when someone else is in a better position to do so. For instance, a dental hygienist might be the most appropriate person to count the frequency of disruptive behavior by a patient in the dental chair; or the spouse or parent can be asked to count the toothbrushing behavior of another family member.

To facilitate the comparison between baseline counts and the counts taken after the change or intervention procedure is initiated,

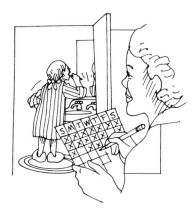

the counts are expressed as **rates** or **baserates.** The rate at which any activity or event occurs is the number of times it occurs during a given period. For example, when we say a behavior occurs once a week, eight times a minute, or six times an hour, we are making statements about the rate at which the behavior occurs.

Counting and Recording Techniques. Once you or your patient begins to collect information, it is important that it be recorded in a simple and efficient manner that will allow you both to see what progress is being made. There are several ways to keep track of behavior. Here are some of the counting and recording techniques most frequently used and the advantages and disadvantages of each.

Event recording. Obviously, the most accurate behavior counts are obtained when behavior is recorded every time it occurs. **Event recording** is simply the process of recording the pinpointed behavior each time it occurs and then expressing the total number of occurrences as the rate of behavior.

Home Care Project

Name _MS. ADAMS_

Objective _BASERATE - 2 WEEKS_

Week	Sun	Mon	Tues	Wed	Thur	Fri	Sat
No. 1 Dates 9/7 to 9/13	B 9AM	B 8AM	B 8AM	B/F 7AM	B/F 7AM	B/F 6:30AM	B 11AM
No. 2 Dates 9/14 to 9/20	B 10AM	B/F 7AM	B 8AM	B/F 7AM	B 8AM	B/F 7AM	B 10AM

Another simple and inexpensive technique involves the use of some small object which can be easily moved from one spot to another each time a behavioral event occurs. For example, coins or paper clips can be moved from one pocket to another. Counting with small objects can also be done when you have to move around, but it can be cumbersome when you are counting a high frequency of behavioral events.

Grocery and golf stroke counters are two counting devices which are obtainable and easy to use. Many people find such mechanical devices ideal for event counting as well as for counting the permanent products of behavior which will be discussed later in this chapter. The disadvantage to mechanical counting devices is that they may be noisy and call attention to the fact that you are counting. However, in self-change projects or in projects with patients, the idea is usually to make the person more aware of his behavior, and counters do this very well.

Time sampling. With some behavior, such as nailbiting or thumbsucking, practical considerations make it difficult or inconvenient to count every instance of behavior twenty-four hours a day. In such cases, it is customary to record events in a way that makes determining the rate as easy as possible. Using **time sampling,** a specific time slot can be selected and the frequency of behavior counted for the same amount of time each day.

Time sampling works in the same way as event recording except that by using time sampling procedures you make it unnecessary to observe an individual or group of individuals continuously. By specifying what time period or situation you intend to count, you make it unnecessary to count throughout the day. For example, a parent may decide to count instances of thumbsucking between 10 AM and 12:30 PM and between 4 PM and 5:30 PM each day. Thus, as in event recording, you count every instance of a behavior, but only for a specific period of time.

Counting the permanent products of behavior. The **permanent products** method can be used whenever a pinpointed behavior results in a concrete product which can be counted: for instance, the number of cigarettes left in an ashtray, or the number of assignments completed in class. When you use the permanent products method of counting, counts can be taken once a day or once a week and recorded as daily or weekly rates. When you are counting the behavior of another, this method of counting frees you from the necessity of being present whenever a behavior is exhibited.

In summary, counting is the skill of determining the frequency with which a pinpointed behavior occurs during a given time.

Steps Toward Behavioral Change

Some Methodological Considerations. We believe it is desirable to have a person count his own behavior, because counting tends to focus a person's awareness on the specific behavior which he may ordinarily exhibit or fail to exhibit through habit or oversight. However, it is important to note that when a person is taking baseline data on himself, or on another person who is aware that his behavior is being recorded, the behavior being recorded will tend to either decrease or increase in frequency, depending on the desired results. In other words, *baseline recording tends to affect the rate of behavior when the individual is aware recording is taking place.* For example, when a person begins recording the number of cigarettes he smokes each day, it is not surprising that the number drops off day by day. Counting can often be an effective method of getting a person to change his behavior by just increasing his awareness of it. Thus, in situations where the person is aware of baseline counting, *it is important that the baseline period be long enough to obtain an accurate count before the formal intervention plan is begun.*

There are some situations where baseline counting can be done without the individual's awareness, such as when a parent records a child's toothbrushing frequency. Then what is called a 'true' preintervention baseline can be obtained.

How long should you take baseline counts? Baseline counts of behavior are usually taken for 5 to 14 days before implementing a change procedure. This observation period provides you with a pretty good idea of a behavior's frequency and enables you to decide what you'd like to see happen to that behavior and to set reachable goals. A 5- to 14-day baseline also gives you an opportunity to address any problems that may arise in counting. For example, you may discover that your counting method is too obtrusive or too inconvenient.

Even though you will find yourself eager to begin the change procedure, it is extremely important not to skimp on baseline counts. A

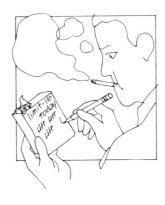

major reason for the failure of many projects lies in insufficient baseline counting. If you don't have a clear idea of what a behavior is like before you try to change it, how can you evaluate the effectiveness of your change procedures and correct any mistakes you might be making? Even short baselines are probably better than no baseline at all.

Charting Baseline Data

As the baseline data are collected, they need to be placed into chart form. Charts enable the viewer to tell at a glance what is happening to the particular behavior over a definite period of time. The following charts offer a visual representation of a particular behavior and its frequency over a specific period of time.

As you can see from chart 1, the baseline period was one week. In chart 2 you will note that the frequency of the behavior has been recorded as treatment time per session with a fearful child. The vertical axis of the chart is always used to represent behavior frequency, the horizontal axis to record the time period.

Keeping a Diary

Up to this point, we have talked only about baseline data gathering in terms of frequency or rate. There is another aspect of this process which is very useful when a patient is trying to modify his own behavior outside the dental office. Besides simply recording the frequency of action or nonaction, he can also record the number of times he thought of the behavior—for example, the number of times he thought of smoking but resisted it, or the number of times he remembered to brush, but did not do so.

We believe that it is important that a patient also record, in a log or diary, how he felt at the time of the recorded behavior. Obtaining subjective feelings and impressions can help you achieve success in a project by telling you more about how the patient really feels about what he is doing. The following examples were collected by our students who attempted to help friends and patients stop smoking.

"I know this is supposed to just be the baseline period, but when I saw that I'd already smoked ten cigarettes and it wasn't even 11 AM, I just put the pack back in my pocket."
"It's too hard to write down every time I do this."
"It really feels good to have a cigarette after breakfast."

Comments about the thoroughness of home care activities may be revealing. For example, "I finally had time to do a good job." "I feel

Steps Toward Behavioral Change

Chart 1

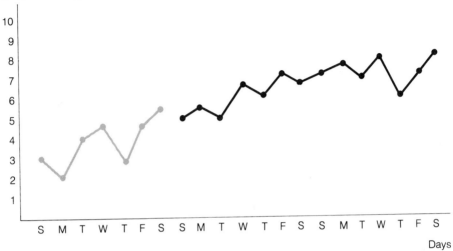

Number of Hours
of Headgear Wearing

Chart 2

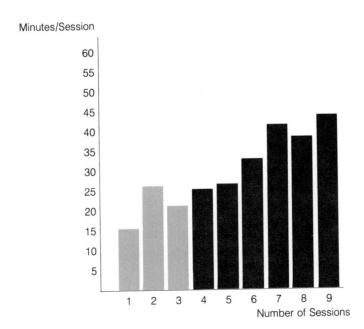

Planning to Collect Baseline Data

like I'm just going through the motions." "At least my breath smells O.K." Such information may prove vital in helping you design a realistic project that has a greater chance of success.

The Baserate Contract

A technique which you may use to help solidify any agreement with a patient is to write up a **contract**, giving a copy to your patient and retaining one for yourself. Perhaps it is because we are such a legalistic, document-oriented society that a contract, which is no more than a written statement of what you have both agreed to do, seems to make it 'more real' or 'official'. Patients are more careful in saying what they will do when they know the results of the discussion will be written into a contract. When agreement is reached, patients will take the written commitment seriously and will usually attempt to live up to their end of the agreement. Unfortunately, verbal agreement, though better than nodding or passive acquiescence, is not as powerful. Moreover, contracts also serve as a reminder of the original agreement.

This is not to say that a contract cannot be changed—it should always be open to modification. But any change should be a result of a discussion between the two of you. Contracts are most often used (1) to help clarify agreements to collect baseline information, and (2) in specifying the conditions of the intervention plan once baseline data are collected and the goals of the program are agreed upon.

In Assignment II of your project, there is an example of a baserate contract that illustrates how contracts may be used. It is important to remember that a contract is a technique that can be used to help both you and the individual you are working with to specify exactly *what* you want to accomplish and *how* it will be accomplished. It is not a tool to browbeat the patient into doing what you want him to do.

With the presentation and negotiation of the baserate contract, thus ends what you can accomplish in the first session. Between the first session and the next time you see the patient, the patient should be collecting baseline data and keeping a log of feelings. During the second session, you will use the baseline information to formulate a specific intervention plan.

A few words about presenting baserates, contracts, or other steps of the behavior change process to another individual are in order at this point. In presenting the idea of baserates or contracts, it is important that your presentation be made in a confident manner. That is, mumbling something like "I'm reading this book and I decided you're going to be a guinea pig," or "I learned this stuff once in a class," will serve only as a prophecy (albeit self-fulfilling) of your own failure. There is, of course, nothing wrong with mentioning that the techniques are new to you—if you convey that you are interested in the patient and your primary goal is to help him change the care he gives his mouth. The techniques and methods you use are merely tools to help facilitate this change.

Your Practice Project
Second Assignment

It is now time to specify the project you would like to work on for the remainder of the book. This assignment consists of two parts: A, outlining a project you will use (or later modify) as the basis of an agreement between you and your patient in which you will identify intervention strategies and potential problem areas; and B, drawing up a baserate contract.

A. Your project outline should include the following five points.

1. Identification of the specific person with whom you will be working and a description of the problem (preferably a management deficiency problem).

   Example 1: The patient is a 26-year-old woman with a parafunctional habit that she believes is detrimental to her teeth and their appearance. She is an elementary school teacher, who, when under stress, often resorts to biting her fingernails as an unconscious reaction to a given situation. The result is excessive incisal wear on #8 that is becoming unesthetic.

   Example 2: The patient is a 20-year-old man who says he brushes almost every day and flosses "once in a while." Because of his repeated pattern of caries, he is concerned about his dental health, that is, 'pink tooth brush', and seems to desire to work with us. He has demonstrated that he can brush and floss correctly.

2. Identification of the method you think you will use to count and record baseline data (for sample recording chart, see page 13).

   Example 1: 3 × 5 card will be carried with patient at all times; data to be recorded in half-hour intervals for one week.

   Example 2: 3 × 5 card will be attached to bathroom mirror; data to be recorded immediately after brushing and/or flossing for a period of two weeks.

For some behavior projects, of course, such as starting an exercise program, the baseline might be zero or close to it. In such cases, this information should still be noted and recorded.

3. Identifying goals. These must be considered tentative, as you will not be ready to set specific objectives until you review the baseline data with the patient. It is important, however, to have an overall view of the project. Therefore, you should:

    a. List a number of possible intermediate goals.
    b. Provide a range of possible ultimate goals.

    Note: Goal statements should be worded positively, as they focus attention on the new habits you wish to establish.

    Example: Intermediate goals—Increase awareness of nailbiting habits and decrease nailbiting by half over the next 3 weeks; or decrease by half over the next 6 weeks; or perhaps increase frequency of using a nailclipper by 50% in 3 or 6 weeks. Ultimate goal—Complete extermination of nailbiting habit or always use nailclippers instead of biting nails.

4. Establish a very tentative time line for the project.

    Example: Baserate—Count for 1 to 2 weeks; Intermediate Goals—Probably try to achieve in 3 weeks; Ultimate Goal—Shoot for 6 to 8 weeks.

5. Specify tentative intervention techniques that you would consider using. For example, what sort of positive consequences should the person expect to receive for successfully achieving each step? Intervention strategies—what you may do to actually try to change the pinpointed behavior—are the subject of chapter 4.

    Examples: I think charting what I do will be a strong incentive to change—self-fulfillment in knowing I stopped. Better self-image in knowing my nails look better; praise from my fiancé; a dinner and theater date at the achievement of each intermediate goal?

B. Making a formal agreement (Baserate Contract).

Once you have outlined your responses for points 1 through 5, you should be ready to present the idea of a change project to a patient, spouse, or friend. To review: In talking to the patient you discuss what you see as the management problem (we are assuming you have already remediated any skill deficits present), and

Steps Toward Behavioral Change

determine whether the patient perceives that he has (owns) the problem. Depending on how the patient responds, you must be prepared to present, or give up, the idea of formally working with that patient on a change project. If the patient perceives a problem, engage him in a brief discussion of when and where the problematic behavior occurs or does not occur. This conversation will set the stage for making arrangements with the patient for him to collect baseline data. Specify all arrangements in contract form. Contracts can be very useful, both during the baseline and intervention stages of the project. They help commit the person by specifying exactly what will be done and make the project more serious or real.

Following the points presented above, write (type or handprint) a baserate contract. On this page and the next are examples of contracts. Examples of charts are presented on page 23.

Once the patient has agreed to collect baseline data, ask him to keep a daily log. As we previously mentioned, having the patient record not only frequency, but also how he actually feels about what he is doing will give you invaluable clues on his motivation, the difficulties he has, and how best to design the intervention strategies. If you rely on the patient to remember and summarize his experiences, you will get only a very small portion of the valuable information you would obtain from a log consisting of a daily, one- or two-sentence entry — possibly written on the chart itself.

Sample Contract Form for Baserates

I agree to do the following before my next appointment on

_____

1. Post a 3 × 5 monitoring card on the bathroom mirror or wherever I brush/floss.
2. Check off on the monitoring card right after each time I brush/floss for the period beginning _____ and ending _____
3. Write down my feelings and impressions each time I brush/floss, making sure to specify how *thorough* I thought I was.
4. Bring the card to my next appointment.

Date _____   Signed _____

Other Sample Contract Forms

Form 1

We, the undersigned, agree to work together to increase

_____ *

Patient's Responsibilities

1. The patient will participate in the treatment program for his/her problem.
2. The patient will carry out all homework assignments given at the end of each meeting. Examples of these are:
   a. keeping a record of dental care activities;
   b. carrying out specific dental care activities.
3. The patient will attend two subsequently scheduled treatment sessions and one scheduled follow-up session.

Dental Professional's Responsibilities

1. He/she will provide the patient with information regarding the general condition of the patient's mouth.
2. The professional will instruct the patient on how to increase desirable dental health behaviors.
3. The professional will attend all scheduled sessions and monitor the patient's records and improvement.

Date _____ Signed _____

Form 2

I have agreed to do the following before my next appointment on

_____

1. Post my 3 × 5 monitoring card on my bathroom mirror.
2. Brush my teeth every morning and evening.
3. Floss my teeth every night.
4. Check off on my monitoring card each time I brush or floss.

Date _____ Signed _____

* Specify patient goal here, for example, "appropriate nightly flossing."

Assignment II

Charts (Examples)

The two charts you see below are examples of how records can be kept during both the baseline and the intervention periods. Many health professionals have such charts photocopied on pads so that they can hand them out to patients, rather than requesting that patients go home and draw them up for themselves.

Home Care Project

Name_____

Objective_____

Week	Sun	Mon	Tue	Wed	Thur	Fri	Sat
No. 1 Dates ___to___	____	____	____	____	____	____	____
No. 2 Dates ___to___	____	____	____	____	____	____	____

No. Cigarettes Smoked

Date_____

Always do one thing less than you think you can do.
  Bernard Baruch

3 The Third Step

Specifying Goals and Objectives

Once baseline data have been collected, you and your patient will have a clear picture of what has happened—when and where the behavior you wish to change is occurring, or not occurring. In the second session, you will be in a position to discuss establishing goals and objectives for change.

Choosing Long-Term Goals and Intermediate Objectives

We define **goals** as long-term targets. Although they are useful in helping a person focus on what he wants changed and the end result he is working towards, long-term targets such as brushing and flossing after every meal or losing 25 pounds, though reasonable, are remote and not easily achievable within a short period of time. By focusing only on the long-range goals you invite failure.

It is much more practical to focus on measurable **intermediate objectives.** These are intermediate targets, or steps which "come along the way" or build up to your ultimate goal. For example, if you find from the baseline data that your patient is brushing or flossing twice a week, it would be unrealistic to expect the patient to start brushing and flossing every day within a week. The goal requires too radical a change in the patient's behavior and will lead to failure. Similarly, focusing only on the goal of losing 25 pounds ignores the much more crucial process of systematic weight reduction. The intermediate objectives of 1 to 2 pounds per week, or even more specific objectives of consuming only a certain number of calories each day, are measurable and easier to achieve.

It is helpful to state goals and objectives in terms of behavior you want to increase, rather than focusing on stopping or decreasing a behavior. Thus, if a person is concerned about his nailbiting, the goals and objectives might focus on "using my nail clipper whenever I want to trim my nails," rather than stopping nailbiting.

At the same time, both goals and objectives should also be as specific as possible. Achieving "good dental health," for example, is a goal that is too general to be of use. When is "good dental health" achieved? How can it be measured? Such questions help in setting goals and objectives.

It is critical that the intermediate goals that are specified be reachable. The baseline data help you to set realistic objectives. If, for example, baseline data indicate that your patient wears his headgear three hours a day, four hours a day may be a realistic initial intermediate objective. It is easy to be overly optimistic and enthusiastic in setting objectives; however, it is your responsibility to caution the patient to avoid shooting too high. It is much better to set the goals too low initially—setting them too high can invite failure. Successfully reaching an intermediate objective will result in feelings of success and the desire to make additional attempts to achieve the next, slightly more challenging intermediate objective. Failure to reach an intermediate objective that is too difficult to achieve will result in frustration and frequently will jeopardize further attempts. Steady, step-by-step progress from objective to objective is slower than leaping to the ultimate goal in one giant step, but far more likely to achieve satisfactory results.

Counseling patients to set realistic goals is challenging. As success depends upon individualizing a program for each patient, your knowledge of patient baserates and general familiarity with the patient are extremely useful.

What About Individual Differences in Patients

As a health professional, when you help initiate a program to break an old behavior pattern or establish a new one, you are simply using your knowledge of psychology to help people change. When people learn how to effectively change something about themselves, they strengthen and develop an ability which we call in everyday life their willpower. When people fail to successfully guide their own destiny, their stock in themselves goes down and they are less willing to try to change themselves again.

Generally, the younger or less accomplished the patient, the less likely he has developed a facet of willpower or self-direction most of you developed and strengthened over the years. This important facet of willpower is the ability to delay gratification, or put off what is pleasurable now for some future benefit. By going to school and studying, you gave up some immediate pleasures in order to reap career satisfaction and financial rewards in the future. By not breaking study schedules, students will get better grades at the end of the term. A success or an achievement that requires effort and striving to

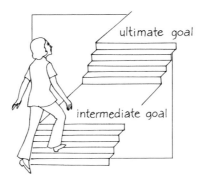

change ourselves strengthens our control over our environment. By the same token, those who have been unsuccessful in controlling their own behavior may see themselves as weak and unable to control themselves or the world around them.

Therefore, though we recommend small steps for everyone, it is especially important to proceed slowly with patients who have not demonstrated an ability to achieve goals they have set for themselves in the past. Paradoxically, when these patients desire the goal, they will usually attempt to reach the goal, if left to their own devices, in one very large step—most often without success. After failing, these patients are unlikely to attempt a small intermediate objective.

The patient's home environment is an important factor. Patients who receive little or no support from family and friends as they attempt to reach objectives are less likely to persevere or to maintain a new behavior over extended periods of time. More moderate goals and objectives may be all that are obtainable. In addition, if you are aware of a significant change in routine or stressful circumstances affecting the patient you may want to resequence or even temporarily delay a step or two until things calm down and the patient returns to a normal routine.

Finally, those who have experience in playing an active role in maintaining their health seem more likely to achieve objectives than those patients who are accustomed to a more passive role. Patients who expect the dentist or physician to "make them well" or to "take care" of them or who are accustomed to regimens which require little or no sustained effort or responsibility on their part are likely to be disappointed by this step-by-step approach, as they are by other approaches which require their active participation.

Where there is the necessary technical skill to move
mountains, there is no need for the faith that
moves mountains.
  E. Hoffer

4 The Fourth Step

Planning an Intervention

Introduction

Chapter 4 is long—but with good reason. Each step has a separate corresponding chapter; thus chapter 4 includes all of the specific strategies and techniques of intervention that we will discuss for establishing new behavior or increasing the frequency of existing behavior, and for decreasing the frequency of problematic behavior. In reading this chapter, keep in mind the project you will do and which of the strategies could be used to achieve your goal.

We suggest that you not try to read this chapter at one sitting. Stop at the end of each section, put the book down for a while, and think about what you have read before starting the next section.

The chapter is divided into five major sections.

Part A: Remediating skill deficiencies—What to do when patients don't know how

1. Modeling
2. Prompting
3. Fading
4. Some methodological considerations

Part B: Remediating management deficiencies—Increasing appropriate behavior by changing antecedents and consequences

1. Antecedents and consequences—How they affect our behavior
2. Identifying antecedents and consequences
3. Using antecedents to change behavior
4. Using consequences to change behavior
   a. Rearranging the sequence of events
   b. Providing positive reinforcers
   c. Applying positive consequences in dentistry
   d. Using tokens
   e. Using reinforcement: four principles
   f. Are rewards ethical

Part C: Remediating management deficiencies—Decreasing inappropriate behavior by changing antecedents and consequences

1. Punishment
2. Altering the chain of events
3. Stimulus control
4. Extinction
5. Incompatible behavior

Part D: Designing a program—Techniques of shaping and charting

Part E: Summary and Assignment III

In session two, you will design an **intervention** plan to change the problem behavior. In helping patients change, it is a good idea to bring as much leverage as possible on the problem. This usually means using more than one technique or procedure to try to change the behavior. You might employ two or even three different strategies simultaneously. The ideas and methods presented in parts B and C may be used in almost any combination to fit the specific individual problems and circumstances. The information provided in part D is important in setting the goals and objectives of any project you design.

Part A Remediating Skill Deficiencies

What to Do When Patients Don't Know How

We said that the most crucial decision you have to make is whether the problem is a result of a skill deficiency or a management deficiency. If the person has a skill deficiency, how do you produce the desired behavior in the first place?

Sometimes all the encouragement or reinforcement in the world would not enable us to suddenly produce desired skills. The problem is this: First you must produce the behavior so that you can encourage it to continue! To begin with, we will focus on the techniques that can be used to establish new behavior patterns. Most of you will be familiar with many of these techniques, as they are part of the health education model of prevention. They are good techniques and effective if the problem is a lack of knowledge or skill.

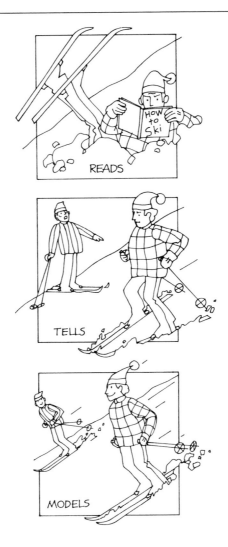

Modeling

You may have seen children play a game called 'monkey see, monkey do', where one youngster does something, like raising his hands over his head, and the other children imitate him. This game illustrates **modeling,** one of the most basic and effective ways to learn new behavior (Bandura, 1969). Did you ever try to learn how to do something you had never tried before by reading about how to do it? You may find you have difficulty even if someone tells you how to do it. Contrast this situation with one in which someone demonstrates or **models** the behavior. Modeling is a very effective way to get someone to do something he has not done before by showing him what the behavior looks like and the consequences that follow the behavior. For example, you are using modeling when you teach a patient how to brush properly by demonstrating on a large plastic model or demonstrating on your own teeth. Audiovisual aids such as filmstrips or handouts may also be helpful in this respect.

Modeling can also be effectively used to reduce the anxiety and inappropriate behavior of fearful young patients. You might invite a shy, withdrawn child who is worried about dental procedures to sit in the room to observe the treatment of a child of the same age who has little fear of the dental appointment and does not mind being watched. Videotapes or films of one's peers undergoing successful dental treatment have also proved useful. In using this kind of modeling it is important that the person perceive the model to be similar to himself. A 4-year-old watching a 13-year-old go through the procedure would probably be minimally influenced.

Prompting

Another common technique used to teach new behavior is called **prompting,** or **cueing.** First, words can be used to help create new behaviors—that is, you can tell someone what to do or provide him with written instructions. Second, gestures can be useful in explaining or calling attention to things. For example, when a child practices brushing, we may prompt him with words and gestures. **Hands-on** prompting can be used to begin instruction in an activity which will be completed independently. A familiar example is the golf pro standing behind the duffer and physically guiding his swing. Instead of merely watching, as when someone else is modeling, the person can feel his body performing the task. With the hands-on technique, the person's body is moved into position physically and he is shown what has to be done. This technique has been very effectively used with young children or retarded patients. When parents are aware of this technique they may easily teach brushing and flossing to their children.

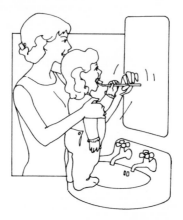

Steps Toward Behavioral Change

Fading

Another procedure, **fading,** involves the gradual removal of such prompts or cues. For example, you may think of training wheels on a bicycle as prompts. When the child first attempts to ride, the bicycle has large training wheels. After the child has learned to ride with large training wheels, smaller wheels are substituted. Eventually, when the child can ride smoothly on small training wheels, these are removed. Fading allows the learner to proceed confidently. Prompts are removed only when the learner is ready. The procedure is based on his rate of learning and helps him minimize physical and psychological bruises that occur when prompts are withdrawn abruptly.

Some Methodological Considerations

Behavior that your patients do not now possess and that they cannot perform must be learned. Some form of modeling is helpful when patients attempt a first approximation of the behavior. Since it is a first try, you should not expect new complex behavior to emerge full-blown or spontaneously. Similarly, once your patients know how to perform the behavior in question, it is perhaps too much to ask that they suddenly start to perform it consistently and religiously.

Providing as many prompts or cues as possible when the person first tries a task facilitates learning. In addition, providing frequent and specific feedback is an important part of the prompting or cueing process for patients. You should pay special attention to the positive aspects of the patient's performance. Moreover, before some patients are able to succeed, you may need to demonstrate proper performance more than once, or to encourage them with positive comments and smiles. Disclosing tablets and inexpensive mouth mirrors are valuable in indicating plaque formation; these items focus on problem areas while minimizing negative verbal feedback that tends to discourage the determination to master new skills.

Though patients may be able to demonstrate adequate skill in the dental office, it is not unusual to find that, without positive feedback from the dental professional, they may not brush or floss properly at home. Why not?

The major difference is that when patients are demonstrating their ability in front of you, they are really trying, actively concentrating on what they are doing. At home they are more likely hurrying, distracted, thinking about what they are going to do or what they did that day. They are not focusing on the task.

There are a number of other factors which may affect the adequacy of home care. In your office patients are practicing with adequate light, hand mirror, and a dry brush so that they can see what they are doing. At home, toothpaste obscures brush positioning; inadequate lighting and bathroom fixtures that block access to mirrors do not help. We recommend that you point out such potential problems to patients, and stress the importance of proper brushing and the futility of improper brushing. Hand mirrors and proper lighting (a stronger bulb) are helpful, as is the banishment of toothpaste until brushing is completed.

Part B   Remediating Management Deficiencies

Increasing Appropriate Behavior by Changing Antecedents and Consequences

There are two principles which underlie all procedures used in changing behavior. The first is that all behavior is learned—any relatively permanent change in a person's behavior occurs because of interaction with the environment. Sometimes learning experiences are structured, as when we go to school or take a continuing education class. Other times learning is a result of trial and error, as when we teach ourselves to ride a bicycle. Learning can also take place unintentionally—we may not even be aware that learning has taken place. For example, as children we eventually learned to let a hot cup of chocolate cool before taking the first sip.

The second principle is closely related—an individual's behavior is a function of his environment. In other words, the behavior a person exhibits in any situation depends a great deal on that situation. For example, we all act differently when we are with patients than when we are among relatives and friends.

Antecedents and Consequences
How They Affect Our Behavior

The circumstances in which we find ourselves clearly influence what we do. These circumstances are:

A. antecedent conditions of the behavior
B. the pinpointed behavior you wish to alter
C. consequences of the behavior

On the basis of thousands of observations and experiments, behavioral scientists have found that the events which have the biggest effect on a behavior are those which occur *just before* the behavior is exhibited (antecedents) and those which occur *just after* (consequences).

By modifying either the antecedents or consequences, we provide a person with new learning experiences and supply new information about what will follow a particular behavior, or the situation in which it is appropriate. For example, when we distract a fearful child, obscure his view of the needle, or tell him to expect a little feeling "like this" (pinch child), we are altering antecedents or what happens before the child responds to the injection. When the child is told he is being a "good helper" in keeping his mouth open wide, we are altering the consequences of responding appropriately to the injection.

Strictly speaking, antecedents and consequences do not cause behavior; however, over a period of time, the repetition of a particular consequence in the presence of a particular behavior results in a very strong connection between behavior and the events surrounding it. Patients who do not receive adequate anesthetic rapidly learn to behave in ways to avoid painful procedures. Also, at times patients who in the past were inadequately anesthetized may learn to report pain even though anesthetic was administered appropriately. However, the truth of the matter is, reports of pain are usually followed by practitioner attempts to reduce the pain.

Some consequences strengthen behavior—that is, they increase the probability the behavior will occur in the future. Other consequences weaken behavior—decrease the probability that the behavior will be repeated. Generally, the consequences immediately following a behavior are considered to be the most important factors influencing the strength of that behavior. Thus, most change procedures emphasize altering consequences.

Most people intuitively recognize that the consequences of today's behavior affect the way we behave tomorrow. This recognition is embodied in the system of rewards and punishment used by families, schools, and business organizations. Even though we usually recognize how much systems influence our behavior, we often forget that we are always providing consequences for other people's behavior, even when we are not handing out reprimands, gold stars, or pay raises. In other words, we are continually teaching people how to behave, often without being aware of what we are doing or of the effect we have on others. If we more often than not run behind on appointment schedules, patients soon learn that ten o'clock really means 10:25, or even 10:40. Every time we praise, ignore, reject, or criticize a patient, chances are that we are teaching that patient something which will affect his future behavior.

We cannot always predict what effect a particular consequence will have, and the consequences which would increase our own behavior may weaken someone else's. Further, the consequences do not always have the effect we desire, and the effect may in fact be opposite from what we intended. For example, it is not uncommon to find that a good bawling out or a spanking may increase the likelihood that a child will repeat the behavior for which he was reprimanded. In such instances, punishment seems, from the neglected child's viewpoint, to be a desirable consequence because the child can only attract parental attention by misbehaving.

It is important to remember that consequences affect the likelihood of a behavior happening because the individual himself finds the consequence that follows either desirable or undesirable.

Identifying Antecedents and Consequences

Identifying the observable antecedents and consequences of a behavior or habit can go a long way towards facilitating change. By identifying and changing these events, we can significantly affect the strength of that behavior in a relatively short period of time.

The best time to look for the antecedents and consequences is when you or your patient are taking baseline counts of a behavior. For example, though your patient might try very hard to change, the situations in which he finds himself may make it all but impossible to successfully change. Obstacles that interfere with what your patients want to do are often present. A patient may find that no matter how much earlier she gets up in the morning, there is always one more thing to do to help the children get off to school—there is never enough time to brush. Other people may also get in the way. In some households, there may be a lineup every morning in front of the bathroom. In such circumstances, the conscientious individual who desires to brush and floss may, in fact, be punished for his conscientiousness.

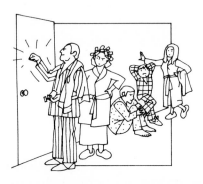

Identifying and eliminating, or minimizing such obstacles may be all that is needed to provide a clear path to change. An effective intervention in such a situation would involve helping the patient find a better time and/or place to brush and floss so that these activities would not interfere with the activities of others or cause their wrath.

In some respects, observing antecedents and consequences is as much an art as it is a skill. The more experience you have with a particular patient, or with a particular problem, the more adept you will become at discovering what types of events exert the most important influence on the behavior in question.

There will be times, of course, when the events which control a behavior are not observable. For example, a person's own thoughts may sometimes be the most significant antecedent or consequence of a particular behavior—or the specific antecedents and consequences controlling a behavior may not always occur in the same situation in which the behavior occurs. If you cannot identify the antecedents or consequences which consistently surround the behavior you wish to change, these events are probably not observable. However, this does not mean that you cannot proceed with behavior change programs. The antecedents and consequences that you provide the patient in modifying behavior will be observable and countable, and you will be able to assess their effects on the behavior.

Using Antecedents to Change Behavior

Antecedent events affect behavior not because they are desirable or undesirable in themselves, but because through experience the antecedents have become associated with particular consequences. Antecedents can best be thought of as **cues** or signals that a particular behavior will be followed by a particular type of consequence. For example, to a motorist, the sight of a police car is a cue that the consequence of his speeding will be ticketing by the patrolman. To many people, the sight or smell of food—or the very thought that there is a goody in the refrigerator—may be a cue to snack.

As we learn to associate certain types of consequences with certain behavior, the antecedent situations that are the cues to those consequences come to exert a powerful effect on behavior. When a motorist spots a police car (the cue), his response to slow down is automatic—it almost seems as if the sight of the police car causes him to reduce his speed. Similarly, without saying anything, the approach of the dental practitioner often causes patients to open their mouths wide.

Rearranging and controlling antecedents can be of use in the dental office. Even time may be used as a cue. For example, a child may be shown an egg timer and told that if he sits still in the chair for ten minutes he will be able to play with the toys in the waiting room while the dentist goes off and performs other duties. This structuring of time may prove useful for anxious adult patients. Such structuring of the dental appointment allows the anxious patient to pace himself. For example, the knowledge itself that discomfort will be only for fifteen minutes and that there are only seven minutes left before the procedure ends or a break occurs can be very helpful for this type of patient.

As we mentioned previously, when you collect baseline information, it is helpful to determine the frequency of the behavior and to describe circumstances surrounding it. When helping a patient establish a regular oral hygiene habit, you may find that there is no time pressure or other interference, but that the toothpaste, brush, and especially the floss may be kept in the medicine chest, 'out of sight and out of mind. In such a situation, no antecedent cues to brush or floss are apparent. It is not always necessary to make wholesale changes in the antecedent situation. At times all that is necessary is to arrange for an antecedent cue to occur regularly in order to help remind the person to perform the desired behavior. Placing the toothpaste or floss in a highly visible place provides a cue for the behavior you are trying to increase. Taping a monitoring chart to the bathroom mirror may also serve as a very strong reminder. Such cues help us by triggering our memory (or by not allowing us to conveniently 'forget'). We also believe cues need to be changed regularly—the same cues seen every day may soon be overlooked or ignored.

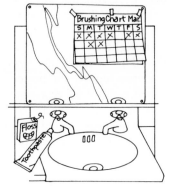

Using Consequences to Change Behavior

Changing the consequences of an event is the most common way of altering behavior. When we reprimand a child, give an employee a raise, thank someone for helping us, or give a student an "A," we are using the system of rewards and punishments to provide feedback which we hope will alter future performance in the direction that is desired. This change is the essence of the reward and punishment system. When we attempt to alter behavior by rewarding desired behavior, we are trying to provide positive feedback that is strong enough to encourage similar behavior in the future.

Rearranging the Sequence of Events. Altering the consequences of an event by using reinforcers or punishment is an extremely effective way to change what people do. Before discussing how such rewards and punishments can be used in dentistry, we will describe how behavior can be increased by simply rearranging the sequence of behavior. This strategy is related to what is called the **Premack Principle,** named after the psychologist who studied the phenomenon.

To help themselves remember how this principle works many people think of it as **Grandma's Law.** The wise grandparent says: "First you clean up your plate, then you can have your dessert." Any behavior that has a higher probabiltiy of being performed (eating dessert) can be used to reinforce any behavior of lower probability (eating vegetables) by making it depend on performance of the less frequent behavior. For example, though most people shower or wash their face every morning, they are less likely to brush or floss their teeth. If you want to increase the probability of a patient's attention to these home care behaviors, you could do so by arranging events so that bathing or washing is dependent upon first brushing and flossing—that is, making an agreement that the patient will not bathe until he brushes and flosses. Here, washing or bathing is more frequent behavior, oral hygiene is the less frequent behavior. Similarly, if a patient always brushes, you would recommend that the patient floss before he brushes.

In using Grandma's Law, we are altering the sequence of existing events and reinforcers. Anything we normally do on a frequent, consistent basis is reinforcing in some way. Reinforcing events often occur naturally, and it is not always necessary to find new reinforcers in order to strengthen a particular behavior. A further illustration:

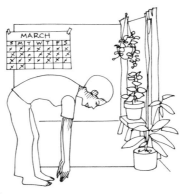

A young woman wanted to increase her exercise time to 15 minutes a day. A very frequent behavior for her was caring for her plants. She simply arranged events so that she could not care for her plants until she had done her exercises.

Students often make use of this strategy when they tell themselves that if they study all day Saturday, they will allow themselves to go out Saturday evening.

The use of this strategy can be especially effective when we try to establish patients' permanent home care habits. We are in effect linking together the new habit we wish to establish with an already existing habit that the patient regularly performs.

The strategy can also be used to identify activity reinforcers to bring desirable behavior under control. Grandma always gives dessert *after* the vegetables and liver are eaten. With a child who seems to have difficulty sitting still in the chair, instead of threatening or criticizing the child verbally, you might make an arrangement for him to have some playtime for a specific time after he has cooperated for a specified period.

Providing Positive Reinforcers. What kind of reinforcers should you use? Since everyone is different, it is impossible to predict exactly what kind of positive feedback or reward will be strong enough to bring about change in a given patient. Let's first look at some basic principles in choosing reinforcers.

1. The reinforcer has to have positive consequences for the individual seeking to change. You should never forget that, no matter how reinforcing the consequence seems to you, it cannot be considered a reinforcer unless it increases the behavior which it follows. People differ and the reinforcers must have value to the person attempting to change and thus must be tailored to suit individual needs and desires.

2. Reinforcers must be relatively strong. The more potent the reinforcer, the more likely it is to help change a behavior. One word of warning: It is our experience that patients can best choose what type of positive feedback will help them change; however, adults are at first likely to choose weak reinforcers, such as an extra half hour of TV or some sort of 'crackerjack' prize. Encourage the patient to choose consequences rewarding enough to alter his current behavior.

For instance: You are helping someone change behavior by altering consequences. Perhaps the person is concerned about brushing, flossing, or wearing headgear regularly. Unfortunately, although the long-range consequences for these kinds of behavior are positive, the immediate consequences are not very strong. And, as we mentioned before, it is very difficult to establish a new habit merely because it is good for you or because it has some other long-range effect. Thus, to increase your chances of success in establishing these new habits, it is wise to provide strong positive consequences (or reinforcers) until the new behaviors become strong enough to maintain themselves without external reinforcements.

The easiest way to evaluate the strength or potency of the reinforcer is to ask, "Does the person seeking to change really think that he will change just because of receiving this reinforcer?" Changing behavior requires work and effort, and most of us, when it comes down to it, are unwilling to work for a pittance.

3. Reinforcers must be accessible. You must be sure that any reinforcer you or your patient selects can actually be delivered. There is no point in cataloguing a hundred dollars as an effective reinforcer if you cannot arrange to collect and give the money. You will be able to tell if a particular reinforcer is accessible simply by asking, "How will the reinforcer be delivered when the desired behavior has been performed?" If you choose a reinforcer which is not available for immediate delivery after the behavior occurs, the effectiveness of that reinforcer will be greatly diminished.

4. Any reinforcement procedure that is selected should be observable. Delivery of reinforcement, just as behavior frequency, should be able to be counted and monitored. Kind thoughts are no substitute for observable reinforcers.

Applying Positive Consequences in Dentistry. How do you go about selecting and choosing reinforcers in dental practice? The list of possible reinforcers is infinite. For a list of suggestions that you may show patients, see Appendix B. In identifying the reinforcers which might be appropriate for a particular person in a given situation, you will find it useful to consider three types of reinforcers: material, activity, and social.

Material reinforcers. A **material reinforcer** is any tangible item you give a person following the occurrence of the behavior which you want to strengthen—such things as food, toys, clothes, jewelry, or recreation equipment.

Activity reinforcers. An **activity reinforcer** is anything a person likes to do. The list of potential reinforcers is also infinite and highly individualized, and includes such activities as watching TV, playing a game, participating in a decision-making process, talking with friends, or taking a walk—any activity which is enjoyed by the person being reinforced.

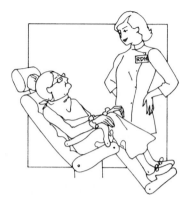

Social reinforcers. Social reinforcement can be thought of as any aspect of one person's behavior which follows someone else's behavior and strengthens it. The most common form of social reinforcement is verbal praise, such as saying to your 8-year-old patient, "Judy, you are being a very good helper by sitting back in the chair like that. You are doing very well," or saying, "Ms. Domoto, three of the patients commented on how quickly you came to help them. I thought you would like to know." Hugging and other forms of physical contact should also be thought of as social reinforcement and may be appropriate to use with children.

Social reinforcement is the most available, and in many ways the most effective, type of positive consequence or reinforcer. In addition to verbal praise, social reinforcement consists of anything you do or say to make a person feel appreciated, accepted, important, or just plain good. Approval, attention, and recognition in any form are usually reinforcing. Simply taking a few extra minutes of clinic time to listen to someone and indicating that you have heard and understood what has been said can be reinforcing.

Because any form of attention may be reinforcing you have to be careful not to reinforce inappropriate or undesirable behavior by the use of criticism. After all, criticism is one form of attention. Criticism is especially likely to reinforce behavior in those homes, schools, or offices where busy parents, teachers, or clinicians tend to notice an individual only when he is exhibiting an inappropriate or annoying behavior. By focusing attention only when someone is exhibiting an inappropriate behavior, we may actually strengthen this behavior. Appropriate or desirable behavior which is ignored is simultaneously weakened.

One form of social reinforcement which is quite effective is **feedback**—that is, simply letting a person know how he is doing, and giving him information about how well he is performing in terms of a specific goal. Feedback is like a mouth mirror or disclosing tablet that shows a person the quality of his brushing. Providing verbal praise to patients during a long procedure, for example, or telling them how they are doing, are ways of increasing the likelihood of cooperation. You might say to your 8-year-old patient, "You're being very good at helping me today by sitting so quietly when I'm looking at your teeth." To an adult patient, you might comment on how much you appreciate his showing up on time for appointments. Notice that these two examples provide the specific information to the patient about what the practitioner found helpful. General social reinforcement or feedback like, "Good," "You are doing just fine," "You are being a perfect patient," can and should be provided occasionally. However, such general comments do not let the patient know exactly what it is you find helpful. It is important to remember that the more specific you can be in providing feedback, the more likely it is that the feedback will have a positive effect on the patient.

Feedback can take many different forms. For children, and even for adults, making a mark on an attractive and well-displayed chart in the home or clinic may itself be reinforcing, even when no other consequences are provided. You may have noticed that towns, hospitals, and charitable organizations trying to raise money often post the current status of their drive, perhaps in the form of a thermometer or a tree sprouting branches, where everyone can see it. People are prompted to do things when they can see their behavior accurately represented in such ways.

Because feedback can be reinforcing, counting and charting of behavior often directly affect the behavior. For example, keeping a record of how many cigarettes you smoke per day or how many times you exercise per week may increase or decrease the behavior in the desired direction. It is important to recall that when a person is aware that baselines are being taken, he is likely to change his behavior—even if he is not yet really trying to do so.

We have seen that social reinforcement may take many forms: recognition, praise, active listening, approval, and verbal or visual feedback. It is important to know about the different forms of social reinforcement because in some situations social reinforcers may be the only ones that are readily accessible. On the other hand, formal recognition of social reinforcement is rarely made in contracts. We health professionals seem uncomfortable in suggesting in writing that approval be made contingent on positive behavior. Moreover, when the behavior of concern is manifested outside the dental office, a family member or friend must be contracted to provide the social reinforcement. We mention these issues because we all need to be aware that providing appropriate social reinforcements at the proper times is a skill that we are not born with, and one that may influence the workability of this kind of intervention.

What kind of reinforcer is it. The distinctions between material, activity, and social reinforcers are not always clear-cut. For example, if a person rewards himself with a certain number of cigarettes at the end of the day for reducing his caloric intake, you might say that the cigarettes are a material reinforcer, or that the opportunity to smoke is an activity reinforcer. (Is it ethical to use cigarettes as a reward? If the individual enjoys smoking, has no intention of giving it up, and is willing to let the habit be the reinforcer, should you impose your feelings?)

Fortunately, it is not really important to categorize the reinforcers that you use to strengthen behavior. The reason for knowing about different types of reinforcers is that it enables you to look at the patient's environment and ask three questions in trying to identify reinforcers. What can I *give* the patient that might be reinforcing? What can I enable him to *do* that might be reinforcing? What can I *say* to him that might be reinforcing?

Using Tokens. Immediate reinforcement is so important that **tokens** are often useful in implementing a reinforcement procedure for adults as well as for children. In situations where you cannot interrupt an ongoing activity to deliver a worthwhile material or activity reinforcer, giving or having someone provide a token (something that can be traded in for some meaningful future reward) can be an effective way to provide feedback and reinforce behavior.

A token can be thought of as anything that can be exchanged for material, activity, and social reinforcers. Physically, a token may be a poker chip, a recorded point, a trading stamp, or a gold star. An example frequently used in talking about token reinforcement is money. Dollar bills have no intrinsic value, but they are valuable because they can be exchanged for material, activity, or even at times for social reinforcers. The use of token systems which do not use real money has proven highly successful in many different settings such as homes, schools, correctional facilities, and hospitals and in work with retarded individuals.

Even with limited funds, you or your patient can use tokens to provide a reward worth working for, for example, an expensive tennis racket, a fancy dress or other item of clothing, time off from a task or job, or a weekend vacation. With the use of tokens we may now deliver down payments for future rewards in situations where no reward or only weak rewards were previously possible.

Material and activity reinforcers can more easily be written into a formal contract than can social reinforcers. However, here too you must rely on another family member or the patient himself to dispense the rewards at the proper time.

Using Reinforcement: Four Principles. There are four basic principles you should keep in mind in designing a program to increase behavior by using reinforcement.

1. When you have a choice of several different reinforcers, you should generally begin by using the one which least disrupts the normal flow of activities and interactions and the one which requires the least amount of intervention. Usually this involves using social reinforcement, which ordinarily consists of some form of verbal praise or nonverbal recognition. It is often the most convenient type of reinforcer to deliver.

2. When you do use material or activity reinforcers, you should also accompany the delivery of these reinforcers with some form of social reinforcement—that is, saying or doing something which demonstrates your recognition or approval. Using social reinforcers with other types of reinforcers is important for any behavior change project. It is really your ultimate goal to bring desirable behavior under the influence of social reinforcement and to eliminate the use of other types of reinforcers, especially material ones. However, material and activity reinforcers are often necessary in the beginning phases of a behavior change project, and they may continue to be the best method of reinforcement for young and retarded persons.

3. Be completely open with everyone about what you are doing. After you have taken your initial baseline counts of the behavior, you and the person that you are working with should negotiate the reinforcement system, the plan of intervention, and the ultimate and intermediate objectives that you are trying to achieve.

4. The contract or agreement that results from this discussion should be open to further change and should not be considered ironclad. At first, reinforcement should occur all of the time, following every instance of the behavior you wish to change. Known as **continuous reinforcement,** this technique is especially important when you are beginning to establish a new behavior, or in instances where the individual whose behavior you are modifying is not fully aware of the consequences, perhaps because he is too young or mentally retarded. In addition, the more immediate the reward, the more likely that it will have an effect. This is true no matter what kind of learning is taking place. If a golf pro watched you practice your swing but waited a week before providing feedback, its value in helping you improve your swing would be greatly decreased. Similarly, when rewards are used by patients to help establish a flossing habit, they should be given immediately after each flossing. Having the parent praise the child's brushing behavior while he is performing it is another example.

Are Rewards Ethical. At this point, you may be wondering if it is ethical to use rewards to get people to do something.

Although people generally accept the idea that it makes logical sense to break tasks down into identifiable steps, accomplish them one step at a time, and keep track of progress, they sometimes balk at the idea of arranging positive consequences or rewarding themselves or others for their progress. They find themselves saying a version of "After all, they 'oughta wanna' do it because it's good for them," or, "We're not going to bribe anyone for doing what he should do in the first place."

Does arranging positive consequences for one's own or for another's performance constitute bribery? Let us look at Webster's definition of bribe. It is ". . . a gift or favor . . . promised with a view to . . . corrupt the conduct . . . of a person in a position of trust . . . ." We are sure that you would be upset if someone suggested that you were trying to persuade patients to do something corrupt.

The eventual goal of any behavior change program is to wean the child or adult patient from externally provided consequences to the intrinsic reinforcements that the successful completion of a task brings. Generally, external reinforcers that the person gives himself, or that you provide, are simply an initial, temporary step.

However, there are some types of tasks that we all perform for which we always expect some external reward. Wages, for example, are contingent on the work we accomplish, and we certainly don't consider ourselves bribed by our employer. In fact, a very common complaint among employees is that they feel that they deserve a higher wage.

Looking at this issue from another perspective, if we were promised that we would receive a million dollars in 25 years, but nothing before the 25th year, how much effect would this have on our behavior? Would we work 25 years for nothing, even though we were to receive a million dollars after the 25th year? We believe that when we provide incentive and motivation for young children or adults to engage in an appropriate activity it certainly is not a bribe. Behavior management systems are simply arrangements to help individuals meet goals by recognizing and rewarding the efforts they make.

For example, the extra bedtime story a parent reads each time his child masters a new skill encourages him to work toward his goal, and provides feedback on his performance. However, such external reinforcers are designed only to be used in the initial stage of a behavior change program. They help provide incentive to a child or adult who has had either little success in changing himself or has not developed internal rewards for the behavior pattern in question.

If you expect a person to perform, it helps initially to provide external consequences that have value for him. Once he begins to experience success and the positive consequences of the behavior itself, the intrinsic, more naturally occurring reinforcers begin to create their own motivation. For example, a parent might arrange some special positive consequence for his child, such as their watching television together, or playing a game, if the child keeps his room picked up. As the child begins to realize the more subtle positive consequences of a neat room, such as being able to find what he wants and the decreased likelihood that things he treasures will be lost, stepped on, or broken, the original externally provided consequence becomes less and less important as the new habit is established.

In summary, providing rewards as consequences is one of the most commonly employed methods to change behavior. Rewarding someone for doing right is not a bribe, but simply recognition and encouragement to continue.

Part C   Remediating Management Deficiencies

Decreasing Inappropriate Behavior by Changing Antecedents and Consequences

We have discussed the effects of altering antecedent events and using positive consequences to increase the frequency of existing behavior. Now we can focus on the fundamental strategies designed to decrease the frequency of existing behavior.

Punishment

The first procedure we will discuss is the most familiar—**punishment.** Let's consider for a moment the concepts of punishment and reinforcement. Both are consequences that follow and change the frequency of behavior. The important difference is that reinforcement increases or maintains behavior, while a punishment decreases or inhibits behavior.

It is important to realize that exactly the same event may function as a punishment to one person and as a reinforcement to another. We have all been tickled at one time or another, some of us enjoy it, some do not. Some times a person likes to be tickled, other times the same person does not. It can be either punishing or reinforcing.

There is no absolute way of foretelling whether a consequence following a behavior will function as a punishment or as a reinforcement. To determine this you first have to record a baseline count of the behavior and then see how it is affected by the consequence. By comparing the baseline record with the behavior after you have presented the consequence, you will be able to see if the behavior decreases or increases in frequency.

Besides suppressing the behavior in question, punishment has a number of unpleasant side effects. First, we find that punishment often results in additional negative behaviors. Anger and uncooperativeness are typical responses. Second, it is frequently seen that when possible, an individual will simply avoid the person applying the punishment. And third, we find that the punished person may be momentarily confused and less able to function effectively. More likely than not, punishment is a technique inappropriate for health professionals.

On the other hand, what can be done on those rare occasions when you find yourself face to face with a child who not only misbehaves during a dental emergency and makes it impossible to proceed with dental procedures, but who also poses a threat to his own physical safety? In such situations, after attempting to get the child to hear you by repeating your orders in a voice with increasing authority, it may be necessary for the child's own safety to employ stern procedures to reestablish communication with him. This is an extremely important point: It is critical to gain the child's attention and reestablish communication.

We believe the use of various physical restraints may be warranted. Restraint may involve pushing down a hand lifted inadvertently or intentionally. During a restorative procedure, for example, it may involve placing a hand over the child's mouth while assistants hold flailing arms and legs. Once quieted down, the removal of the hand is followed by praise and other social and material reinforcements. Used properly, these procedures may rapidly restore communication.

Is the use of physical restraints punishment? Physical restraint can be used as punishment for "bad" behavior such as whining or crying. However, its use as punishment is an abuse of the procedure. Restraints should never be used vindictively. If you feel angry and tempted to use these techniques to win a point or to physically force the child to comply with your wishes, you have lost control of the situation (and your own emotions). Better to end the session prematurely and/or refer the child to another practitioner than to traumatize the child and create negative attitudes toward dental care.

In addition, it is important to note that restraints should not be used for extremely fearful children, for mentally retarded persons, or for extremely young children who are not yet able to communicate and cooperate. It is most effective with children 3 to 6 years of age.

There is one caveat in using this technique that is worth emphasizing—you must be sure you are in complete control of your own emotions. You should not show anger or display annoyance at the child. You must be as matter-of-fact and unemotional as possible. Failure to do so may result in improper behavior management, defeat your own purpose, and do damage to the child. In an article published in 1974, Dr. Levitas, an experienced pedodontist, described the details of the hand-over-mouth approach.

I place my hand over the child's mouth to muffle the noise. I bring my face close to his and talk directly into his ear. "If you want me to take my hand away you must stop screaming and kicking and listen to me. I only want to talk to you and look at your teeth."

After a few seconds, this is repeated and I add, "Are you ready for me to remove my hand?" Almost invariably, there is a nodding of the head. With a final word of caution to be quiet, the hand is removed . . . . As [the hand] leaves the face there may be another garbled request, "I want my mommy." Immediately the hand is replaced. The admonition to stop screaming is repeated and I add, "You want your mommy? . . . All right, but you *must* be quiet and stop kicking and I'll bring her in as soon as I am finished." . . . While the child is composing himself I begin small talk. As soon as he begins to cooperate I praise him.

Use of Punishment Techniques in Altering Oral Health Care Habits. Can or should punishment procedures be used outside the clinic to change oral health habits? It has been found that intervention plans that rely solely on punishment seldom work, primarily for the following reasons. First, undesired behavior is usually resistant to mild punishment, especially when it is applied after a delay. Punishment is most effective as an intervention when it is administered in large amounts immediately following the behavior. For example, not being allowed to see a movie would in all likelihood be too weak to be effective punishment for not brushing. The second reason for you not to use punishment is that punishment usually results in avoidance of the punishing person and other negative emotional side effects that we mentioned earlier. Third, punishment alone does not teach new or alternate forms of behavior. Punishment often merely temporarily suppresses the behavior that precedes the punishment. Fourth, punishment is generally effective in suppressing a behavior only as long as there is someone around to administer the punishment. Finally, though interventions based only upon self-punishments may be effective, there is a strong chance they may not be enthusiastically followed. Most often, when choosing a punishment, people decide to take away some pleasurable event that is usually available, for example, an evening out or a favorite food. In the end, not all people will really follow through on the agreement.

There are some change projects, however, where punishment by itself can be very effective. Some patients trying to decrease nail or cheek biting have reported that by snapping a rubber band on their wrist when they catch themselves performing the undesired behavior, they can decrease or eliminate the habit very quickly.

Clinical psychologists Nurenberger and Zimmerman have reported an interesting intervention strategy that utilizes punishment. Patients agreed that if they did not achieve their objective they would mail a bank check, previously prepared, to the political or religious organization they hated the most. As with the use of other forms of punishment it is best to use this device with reinforcement. As patients successfully reached their objectives, they rewarded themselves appropriately. Similar procedures have been used by other psychologists. For example, in 1971, in an innovative experiment, clinical psychologist Hall and his associates reported that their patients agreed to tear up dollar bills or contribute twenty-five cents to a charity for each cigarette smoked.

Finally, a word of caution about setting up an intervention plan using punishment where another family member is responsible for punishing that patient for performing or not performing the pinpointed behavior. Make sure that both parties wholeheartedly agree to the conditions and that the terms are carefully written out and signed by each.

Now that we have explored a technique that is used only as a last resort, let us focus on some other strategies and techniques which can be used to decrease or eliminate inappropriate behavior.

Altering the Chain of Events

We have talked about how antecedents can be used to increase behavior. Antecedents can also be used to decrease behavior. At times you may want to change the antecedents which lead up to situations that you or your patients find difficult to handle. Many undesirable behaviors are the result of a fairly long chain of events. For example, snacking may involve going to the supermarket, picking out cariogenic snack foods, placing them in a convenient place, becoming bored or having nothing to do for a minute, moving toward the kitchen, opening the refrigerator or pantry, and finally ingesting the snack. By the time the person reaches the end of the chain of events, the impulse to perform the final, but undesirable, behavior is so strong it is difficult to restrain. This is particularly true for what are known as **consummatory** behaviors—such as eating, smoking, and drinking—where a behavior effects the consumption of the reinforcer, and ends the chain. Such behaviors are very difficult to change.

Though difficult, a number of strategies that involve altering an antecedent event are effective in changing these forms of behavior. The first strategy involves a two-stage process. In the first stage, the person deliberately avoids antecedent situations, such as parties, where he might be strongly tempted to smoke, or dinner engagements where there will be a social obligation to eat a lot of high caloric food. During this stage, each time he successfully avoids a tempting situation he rewards himself generously. In stage two, a person rewards himself for being able to withstand the temptation even when exposed to it, such as withstanding hot apple pie while at the dinner party. Three well-known organizations, Alcoholics Anonymous, Weight Watchers, and TOPS (Take Off Pounds Sensibly), use this strategy. The primary focus of the reinforcement they use is on social and interpersonal relations—the approval, caring, and love of others.

A second strategy is early interruption of the chain of events. Sometimes, by carefully thinking about the chain of events, it is possible to identify an early, weak link in that chain. For example, one way of helping a patient control his snacking behavior would be to encourage him to alter shopping habits. If a goody is not immediately available, its absence enforces a pause—the person must then either go to the store or bake from scratch—which helps break the normal chain of events. Or with children, parents might be encouraged to make use of the principle out of sight, out of mind' and place sugar snacks in nonvisible or difficult-to-get-to locations.

One cannot always avoid being bored, or feeling tense, so it is impossible to eliminate these links in the chain. However, a person can change what he begins to do when he has these feelings.

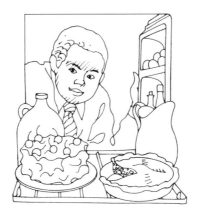

Stimulus Control

Stimulus control is another technique useful for curtailing undesired consummatory behavior, like overeating and smoking. It involves arranging certain situations to provide cues for the behavior one wants to control. Stimulus control and cueing can be used when elimination of the behavior is the goal. The logic is this: If a behavior can be firmly linked to an antecedent, that antecedent can be successively narrowed down in scope to the point where the behavior is unlikely to occur at all. For example, psychologist Nolan reported in 1968 that a smoker agreed to smoke only in her smoking-chair at home. This agreement first brought her smoking under control in a particular place. She no longer smoked at work or when she went out. Once she had established this habit, the chair was placed so that no other reinforcement besides smoking was provided—the chair faced away from the TV set, was not comfortable, and so forth. Once she had established smoking only in this location, she moved the chair out of the living room to the cellar! Under this plan her smoking decreased dramatically.

Similar strategies have been used to control nailbiting and may be techniques that you and your staff might suggest to parents to minimize the ingestion of cariogenic snacks. That is, when children choose to snack, they will agree not to read, talk, watch TV, or engage in any other activity while eating.

Extinction

This strategy is quite different from punishment. Punishment involves presenting negative or unpleasant consequences after a behavior occurs. **Extinction** involves identifying the positive consequences or reinforcements which keep the behavior going and then stopping or withholding these reinforcements or consequences. For example, starting a meeting on time despite the absence of one or two individuals stops reinforcing them for showing up late. If the meeting never starts until they arrive, why should they show up on time? Similarly, when a child misbehaves in a dental chair, calling in the parent prior to completing a procedure will teach the child that misbehaving is a great way to get mom to intervene. Moreover, if the child finds a parent's presence rewarding, episodes of misbehavior will begin to increase.

Typically, the initial results one obtains from applying punishment and extinction are different. When punishment is suddenly begun after every occurrence of a particular behavior, you are likely to see a dramatic but temporary drop-off in that behavior. However, when reinforcement is discontinued, it is not unusual for the person to try even harder to elicit the same reinforcement as before. Thus, if the parent decides to start ignoring the cries of his 3-year-old, or when the practitioner does not stop what he is doing because of the whining of the child, it is quite reasonable to expect that problem behavior will increase temporarily. This phenomenon is called an **extinc-**

tion curve. When using extinction, you must be prepared for this phenomenon and have the patience to wait it out.

Incompatible Behavior

This procedure is similar to simple reinforcement. First you must identify an alternative behavior which cannot be performed at the same time as the undesired behavior. This new behavior is then increased through positive reinforcement to replace or substitute for the undesired behavior. For example, the parents of a 7-year-old who habitually sucked her thumb attempted to reinforce the alternate incompatible behavior of hugging and holding her doll. This procedure is also useful in interrupting the chain of events which leads to an undesirable behavior. For example, instead of moving towards the kitchen a person might 'reach for their mate instead of a plate,' make a phone call to a friend, or chew a piece of sugarless gum.

Experienced clinicians learn to ignore annoying childhood behavior which does not interrupt treatment, such as crying or whining, and to reinforce by praise and other positive consequences all incompatible positive behavior, such as sitting quietly in the chair. Some smokers use the technique of substituting another behavior for smoking. Instead of lighting a cigarette they take a piece of chewing gum. However, mere substitution is rarely adequate. For the person addicted to tobacco, the value of gum compared to tobacco is quite weak. To increase his chance of success in changing, a person should also heavily and quickly reinforce the performance of chewing gum instead of smoking. He might, for example, make an agreement whereby his wife and family verbally compliment him on the progress he is making when he does not smoke, or he might put a quarter into a bank toward a new set of golf clubs as a reward for each time he successfully substitutes gum chewing.

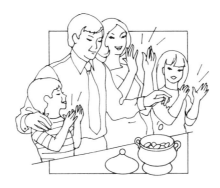

Do not make the mistake of relying only on the mere performance of the incompatible response. An incompatible response must be reinforced—or it will not be continued.

The reinforcement of incompatible behavior is usually a very effective way to eliminate undesired behavior, because you are replacing the undesired behavior with something to substitute in its place. Here is another example of reinforcing incompatible behavior which will further illustrate this procedure.

"Dr. Richman, I'd like to talk to you about my teenage son, Sandy. Though he absolutely hates his dental work, and agrees in principle that it would be a good thing to stop eating sugary snacks, he has not stopped eating the snacks you said cause cavities."

"Did you provide alternate snacks?"

"Both of us shopped for his favorite fruits, nuts, and vegetables. He knows that he shouldn't eat sugar snacks, but that's what he really prefers. When I see him eating that stuff and think of our dental bills, I explode. But that doesn't do any good either."

"Well, simply substituting snacks may not be enough. Do you think you could reward him for eating other foods?"

"Reward him?"

"Yes, instead of trying to convince him that he should prefer healthful snacks, provide praise, approval, and attention when he tries a new snack. You may also want to talk with him about setting up an agreement where you would provide 'special favors' to provide incentive for him till he breaks the junk food habit, which is darn hard to overcome. Want to hear more?"

"You bet."

This illustrates the two techniques that go together: substitution and reinforcement.

Part D   Designing a Program

Techniques of Shaping and Charting

We have discussed techniques that can be used to increase and decrease behavior. Now we can focus more specifically on the actual design of a program and on the use of intermediate objectives and charts during the intervention phase.

Shaping

In chapter 3 when we insisted that it is best to work gradually towards only realistic, reachable intermediate objectives rather than focus on the long-range ultimate goal, we were discussing the concept of **shaping**—the reinforcement of successful approximations in achieving a goal. Shaping is simple and effective when: (1) you begin at the level where the person can succeed; (2) you create intermediate objectives or steps, and reinforce each and every step in the process; and (3) you move step by step in approximating your ultimate goal. For example, if your patients have never flossed, or do not regularly wear headgear or insert dentures, it would be unrealistic to expect substantial changes—especially 100% compliance, during the first weeks of the behavior change program. Starting at their initial level of performance, you need to slowly shape their behavior and abilities.

One of the most common reasons for foundering when attempting to change behavior is the failure to use shaping. Though it is pleasant to think of receiving the positive consequences for immediate accomplishment of the ultimate goal, if you recognize or reward only perfected behavior you will greatly decrease the chance of ever reaching the ultimate goal. You must reward step-by-step approximations that may be much lower than your ultimate goal.

Many people seem to be able to tolerate being an unskilled beginner in a new sports activity. However, there are a large number of people who, after starting a regular exercise program, stop after a brief initial attempt. They may exert themselves beyond their level of endurance in the vain attempt to get in shape, only to find that when they do, they wind up with chest pains and an appreciation of their frailty. People often overdo and push themselves to the limit to get fast results. "If one pill is good for you, then two or three must be better"; "If running is good I'll run till I drop." But results take time, and it is easy to end up feeling "I tried as hard as I could and it didn't do any good."

Similar situations occur frequently in dentistry. Patients with poor hygiene may begin brushing and flossing intensively for a brief period of time. If, in the face of bleeding gums and some pain, they maintain their effort for a week or two, with proper techniques the patients may actually increase their oral health. However, when patients brush intensively, they frequently mistake quantity for quality and may damage oral structures without greatly affecting their oral health. More importantly, they do not begin to build a long-term health care habit. Instead, their efforts are to "get their teeth in shape," a decidedly short-term orientation. The reappearance of symptoms after the intensive efforts have stopped then leads to their thinking that they just have 'bad teeth', or that "it's too much trouble," or "it really doesn't do any good."

Some individuals resist shaping because they believe they should perform at certain levels and do not deserve to take pride in, or be reinforced for, performance below that level. This is an unfortunate attitude, as it removes the possibility of both reinforcement and learning. By the use of shaping techniques, a person begins at whatever level he is currently performing, and slowly but surely moves toward the ultimate goal, reinforcing himself as he progresses. For example, in establishing plaque control for a patient who has never flossed, you should not expect him to be flossing daily within a week. Instead, negotiate and arrange reinforcement for flossing twice a week. Shaping is also used when one is trying to reduce or eliminate a habit like smoking or nailbiting. The statement "To hell with it, I can't do it" is frequently invoked when we lose our willpower. However, such a situation is usually the result of trying to reach our goal too quickly and failing to shape behavior adequately.

There are three simple rules for shaping.

Rule 1: *You can never begin too low.* Whenever you are in doubt, begin at the lower level. If you are having difficulty mastering a particular step, then take a step backward. In some instances, the step which you may have decided upon might be too difficult, and you may have to break it up into several smaller steps.

Rule 2: *See that some positive consequences follow the behavior.* In other words, there should be plenty of reinforcement following each successful step.

Rule 3: *Increase the difficulty of what is to be done—gradually, slowly, steadily.* Almost any program that calls for increasing some desired behavior should have a shaping schedule built into it. The following are two examples which utilize shaping techniques.

Example 1: [Baseline:]"I am now studying approximately four hours per week. This should be easy to do because I have done it before in the past. Level 2: The second week I will require myself to study six hours in order to get the weekly reinforcement. The third week my goal is to study nine hours, and I get the reinforcement only after I have done that much."

Example 2: "From my baseline I see that I am only brushing about four days a week. I almost never manage it on weekends or when I stay up late. For the next two weeks I will try to brush every weekday and at least once on the weekend. I am going to move the time I brush my teeth to the morning. After I reach my goal I will aim for consistent brushing seven days per week."

Notice how carefully the individuals in these examples followed the rules for shaping: start low, keep the steps small. This allows them slow, but inevitable progress.

While it is often tempting to create a time schedule as a motivator, arbitrary calendar dates can retard your progress. Time schedules should be seen only as tentative guidelines. The rule for advancement is: Do not move up a step until the previous criterion is met. The study schedule discussed above has a potential flaw: The student may be tempted to move to level three just because it is week three. He should not do so until level two has been performed successfully.

The Importance of Charting

Whether you are taking baseline data or implementing shaping procedures during the intervention phases of the program it is important to remember to keep good records in chart form. This is important because the records, like a temperature gauge, show you small changes which ordinarily would not be noticed or appreciated. They also serve as an important source of motivation and possible reinforcement for everyone concerned. It is like a daily report card showing successes. For example, a clinician might wish to be able to check the progress of his plaque control programs through a review of the patient's record of the frequency and time he spent brushing, flossing or rinsing. Even though no dramatic changes in the patient's dental problems may occur immediately, the patient can see an objective improvement in his oral health care habits, and the clinician can reinforce these habits. Physicians helping heart and stroke patients and others with needed programs of exercise and diet have used similar shaping and record-keeping procedures to improve self-care activities. Nurses, physical therapists, and others also use shaping procedures to attain goals. For example:

"Mr. Smith, I'm sick of trying to walk. I can't stand the frustration. I am not getting any better than I was."

Compare this conversation with:

"Gee, Mr. Brown, I walked more today than I did yesterday, didn't I?"
  "Yes, you did. You walked 22 steps more according to the charts. You're really moving along."

A good record and chart of improvements serve as measures to detect and appreciate even small improvements in behavior, and can act as a very important source of motivation and reinforcement for all concerned. Using a shaping technique can be very effective in modifying your own behavior, as well as someone else's. In fact, self-control and self-modification procedures depend largely upon the use of shaping and charting skills. If you or a patient wishes to cut down on smoking, you or he can count the number of cigarettes smoked and find the baseline. Then set reasonable goals for reducing the number of cigarettes smoked. Be sure to make a chart, such as the one on page 59, indicating the number of cigarettes you or he smoked each day. Then, change your objectives, little by little, as

Chart 1

Number of Hours
of Headgear Wearing

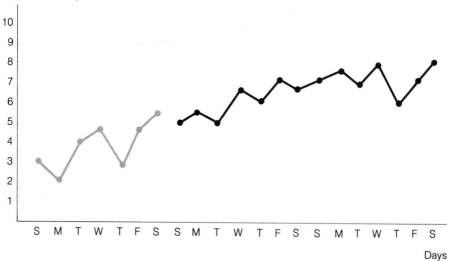

Days

Chart 2

Minutes/Session

Number of Sessions

Steps Toward Behavioral Change

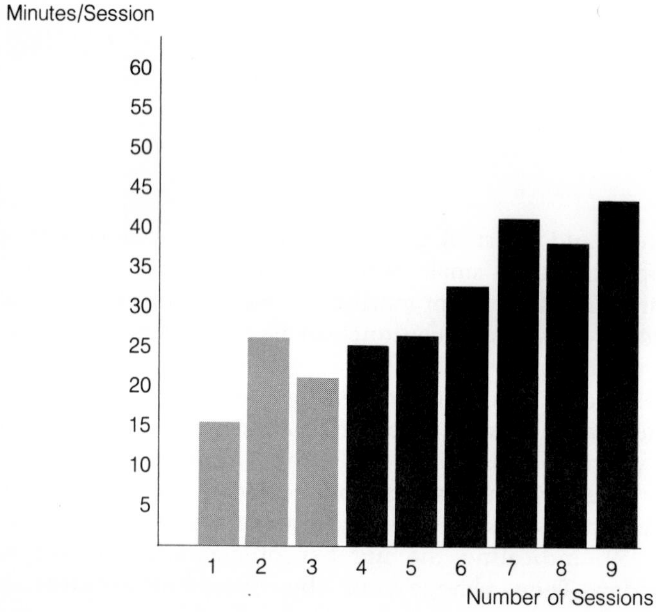

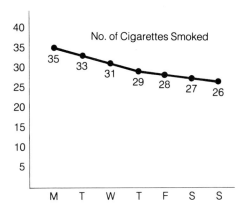

you achieve each objective. The situation is exactly the same when you try to increase the quantity or quality of brushing or flossing or other oral behavior.

When patients attempt such projects, recommend that they place a chart of their brushing, flossing, or other activity in a place where they and others will see it often each day so that relatives and friends can comment on their efforts. Persons desiring to increase the amount of time spent exercising each day often find similar procedures very effective. Marks on the chart, indicating the steps in the exercise program or the number of units spent exercising, will facilitate building up a longer period of exercise each day and provide positive feedback both from the chart and from others.

The Problem of Cheating

Cheating—the delivery of reinforcement without meeting the criteria—is a common problem in self-monitored shaping programs, especially in those which rely primarily on external rewards such as material or activity reinforcers. One solution is for the person to require less of himself by attempting to reach the final goal more slowly.

Cheating, though not a sin, does occur and should be remedied by modifying the intermediate objectives (shaping schedule). Cheating by taking the reinforcer, even though one has not performed the behavior, is fairly common in self-modification. Almost everyone does it sometimes. If your patient is attempting to change his own behavior, you should sensitize him to watch very carefully for cheating.

However, if he cheats more than occasionally, say more than 10% of the time, it indicates a shaping problem. If your patient finds himself in this situation, the progression of intermediate objectives should be redesigned so that he will be reinforced for performing at some level he finds possible.

Part E   Summary and Assignment III

You have (finally) completed chapter 4. You should now be ready to complete Assignment III and present your plan to the patient. Chapters 5 and 6 cover the last two stages of the change process—reviewing and making any modifications necessary, and termination and follow-up of the project.

Your Practice Project
Third Assignment

You have now read the chapters which present specific intervention strategies. With the baseline data that have been collected, you should be ready to choose or suggest a few specific strategies that will facilitate the change that is desired.

As it is wise to bring as much leverage to bear on the problem as possible, we strongly recommend that you choose or suggest combinations of several strategies. This assignment is to help you identify the optimal set of strategies that will work best with the problems presented by your patients. It is common to find that a strategy doesn't work in the way you anticipated it would. Recognizing the problem and what to do about it are discussed in chapter 5.

Once the plan is presented, negotiated, and agreed upon, the particulars of the agreement should immediately be put in contract form outlining (1) the intermediate and final goals, and (2) the intervention strategy and specific conditions of the reward or punishment system used (if any). On the next page you will find a sample intervention contract. In addition, Guidelines for Choosing Reinforcements and a Reinforcement Schedule Survey are included in Appendix B.

Assignment III

The example below will serve as a guide to you for drafting your own contract. Be sure to include possible intermediate and final goals and at least two plausible intervention strategies.

Sample Intervention Contract

I agree to do the following before my next appointment on (date).

1. Continue to post a 3 × 5 monitoring card on the bathroom mirror or wherever I brush/floss.
2. Keep checking off on the monitoring card right after each time I brush/floss for the period beginning (date) and ending (date).
3. Switch the time I usually brush/floss from just before I go to bed to just before I take my shower in the morning.
4. Move the floss canister out of the medicine chest and place it on the bathroom vanity.
5. Place a floss canister on the side table by my favorite chair to serve as a reminder.
6. Keep a daily log (a sentence or two) about how I feel the project is working.
7. My goal will be to brush every day and remember to floss every other day. For every day I floss I will write a check to myself (cash) for one dollar. This money is to go only towards a new metal tennis racket.
8. Bring the card to my next appointment.

Date _____ Signed _____

If something can go wrong, it will.
  Murphy's Law

There is always a wrong solution to every human
problem—neat, plausible, and wrong.
  H. L. Mencken

5 The Fifth Step

Monitoring and Modifying the Plan

We have discussed the first four basic steps in developing a plan to help change your own or someone else's behavior.

Step 1: Identify what behavior you wish to alter, then determine whether it is the result of a skill or a management deficiency. The process of pinpointing is used to discover when and where the behavior in question is occurring or not occurring.

Step 2: Take baseline counts to determine the frequency and rate of the behavior. This serves as a measure against which the success of the change project can be accurately assessed.

Step 3: Specify goals of the project, figuring out specific and realistic intermediate and terminal objectives.

Step 4: Plan and implement what you will do to help change behavior, and specify procedures, objectives, and rewards for successful performance.

In the third session, we focus on the fifth step—monitoring and modifying the intervention plan. Once the intervention plan is initiated, an active watch must be maintained to chart the progress of the program and to work out kinks or trouble spots which occur—and they will occur! It is not at all uncommon that once the program is begun, some unforeseen problem arises which necessitates rethinking and renegotiating an aspect of the project.

What to Do When Little or No Change Occurs

Once you begin the intervention phase, if you are not observing as much change as you expected, or if you do not observe any change after five days or so, there are a number of factors that you might examine—things you can look at as a means of troubleshooting the cause of the problem.

First, *check the counting and reinforcement procedures* that are being used to make sure that you are accurately counting and reinforcing the behavior you are trying to modify. Questions that you might ask yourself include:

1. Am I reasonably sure that the person is counting the behavior as it occurs, and not just estimating its frequency at the end of each day or week? People who estimate are often tempted to discontinue a plan even though it is succeeding, simply because they believe it is failing. The reverse may also occur, and an ineffective plan may be continued for an inordinate period of time. Remember, the best way to organize data for examination is to plot them on a chart or graph.

2. Is the person receiving the reinforcement immediately after he exhibits the appropriate behavior? Timing of reinforcement is important. It is vital in some cases that the reinforcement be provided as soon as possible. This is especially true when you are attempting to vary strong habits. For example, biting your nails, smoking a cigarette, or eating chocolate now feels better than the thought of helping your health or the material or activity reinforcer you will receive next week. By arranging for an extra, immediate reinforcement you can tip the balance toward choice of long-term goals. Praising the smoker when he resists the temptation to light up or the dieter when he turns on the TV after leaving the table without eating seconds is an example.

Second, if you feel this is not the problem area, *consider the nature of the reinforcers.* Some of us are not accustomed to rewarding ourselves or others and initially may opt for only very modest reinforcement. Discuss with the individual whether he feels the reinforcers are strong enough to help change his behavior. Do they really matter enough for the person to make the effort to change? It is very likely that the consequences you are providing for the performance of the behavior are simply not sufficiently reinforcing to the person whose behavior you want to change. While an extra dessert or half an hour of TV time is probably not a strong enough reward to facilitate the reaching of objectives, sporting goods, clothing, jewelry, and weekend vacations or other luxuries will often do the trick. Beefing up the reinforcement can make a real difference. At times, we have found that encouraging a patient to make a down payment or purchase an item on layaway is a useful strategy.

Another common problem is that people often design reward systems on an all-or-nothing basis, where the person has to perform perfectly to receive any reward at all—leaving no room for an occasional backslide or nonperformance. Systems requiring perfect performance are too demanding and usually lead to failure and discouragement on the part of the person trying to change.

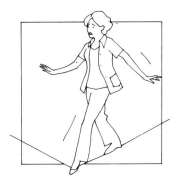

If you are satisfied that the consequences you are providing are as strong as you can make them, and if you are counting and reinforcing the behavior correctly, you should *turn your attention to the environment* in which the behavior is occurring or the environment in which you want the behavior to occur.

There may be a behavior which is currently being reinforced that is incompatible with the behavior you want to alter. This behavior may be reinforced by another person, or by a consequence you have not thought of changing. It is especially difficult to change behavior without the cooperation of spouses, parents, or other family members. For example, a dieter may constantly be pressured by a spouse to attend dinner parties or to eat forbidden foods. Though this problem is not easily solved, sometimes new aids may be restructured so that those significant others' attempt to help and not hinder the behavior change. A weekend for two or an item each really desires may be negotiated into the contract. In another example, a child may keep crying and misbehaving in the clinic even though the hygienist reinforces cooperative behavior with attention and 'TLC'. The behavior continues because the parents or siblings continue to give the child attention for the inappropriate behavior outside of the clinic or office. In such a situation you might use one of several different strategies to eliminate or minimize the interfering behavior. For example, you may desire to structure time for the child, requiring only five minutes of cooperation for a substantial play period, or specific material reinforcer. You might want to work with the parents of the child and instruct them on how to behave appropriately, or even invite them into the operatory. Or you may decide to use the stategy of extinction and simply ignore the inappropriate behavior of the child.

The problem may also lie in the frequency of occurrence of the behavior you wish to increase and reinforce. You may find that the behavior you wish to change may initially occur at such a low rate that there are not many opportunities available for reinforcing it. If you have only two or three opportunities to reinforce the behavior in

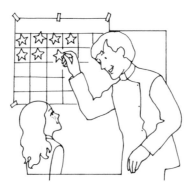

the first five days of the project, you cannot expect to see much change. If an initial low frequency of behavior seems to be the problem, there are two things you can do. First, you may want to increase the likelihood that the behavior will occur by prompting the individual to increase the possibility that he will perform the behavior. For example, you might actually tell the person when it is appropriate to exhibit a particular behavior, and then reinforce it immediately after it occurs. A parent may use such a procedure to help a child develop a brushing habit.

The second thing you can do to increase the likelihood that the behavior will occur is to pinpoint a behavior closely related to the one you wish to alter but which precedes, or occurs more frequently than, the behavior you wish to modify. For example, in order to increase the amount of time a husband spends talking to his wife you might have to first increase the amount of time he spends in the same room with her. Beginning at a lower level of performance than the one you eventually desire is, of course, shaping. Aside from failing to provide strong enough reinforcers, one of the most common reasons for failure in behavior change projects is choosing goals and steps which are too big to accomplish and lead to immediate failure instead of success.

As we mentioned previously, a contract is not an ironclad agreement. As problem situations arise, either from your perspective or the patient's, points of agreement can be reworked and modified to better help you and your patient reach his objectives. As a health professional, your role is to assist in some way to help change a patient's behavior—it is not to make the patient go along with a given plan of goals and objectives. Your flexibility or ability to modify the project will likely be an important factor in its success.

Whatever begins, also ends.
  Seneca

6   The Sixth Step

Terminating the Project

Eliminating the Reward System

As the program progresses and the behavior slowly changes toward the ultimate objective or goal, you must begin to think about terminating the project. The first step in this procedure is the **thinning out** and eventual elimination of any external reward system. As you recall, when the change procedure is first initiated, some kind of reinforcement should follow every time the desired behavior occurs. As the behavior becomes more established, reinforcement should be thinned out. This process can be accomplished in several ways. You might increase the level of performance required to obtain the reinforcement. That is, you might start requiring 100% performance or nonperformance before the reward is received. Or you might set up a schedule where the individual receives a reward, for example, only one time in three. In this case you would not reinforce every third occurrence of the behavior, but instead would scatter reinforcement in an unpredictable fashion to average one reinforcement for every third occurrence of the behavior.

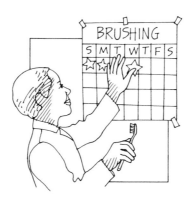

Eliminating the Professional

Concurrently with thinning out the reinforcement, increased responsibility should be given to the individual to monitor or administer the program himself. For a young child, this might mean taking over posting his own gold star on the tooth brushing chart. For an adult, it might mean assuming control of the reward system which was originally handled by his spouse or decreasing the number of checking or monitoring appointments at the dental office. You must be careful to establish this new behavior as firmly as possible in the daily routine of the individual. Remember, the goal is self-maintenance and continuance of the behavior into the future, long after the formal change project ceases.

As the project ends, all external monitoring and reinforcements are generally eliminated. It is easy at this point to find ourselves thinking that the new behavior is established, that we can ease off, or that the change will somehow maintain itself. After all, we wanted it in the first place, and now that we are doing it regularly, why should the behavior fade? Why should we revert to our old pattern?

The fact is that new forms of behavior, no matter how enthusiastic or pleased we find ourselves with the results, are at this point only tentatively established. It is difficult for any new behavior or habit to become second nature, especially if that behavior, like all preventive health habits, has no continuing, immediate pay-off. There is no immediate consequence of failing to exercise today, or eating two pieces of apple pie, or not flossing your teeth.

Follow-Up

Consequently, it is critical that some kind of follow-up be established once the project terminates. One very simple and useful kind of follow-up is the use of monitoring. Individuals often find that it is useful to continue recording the frequency of the new behavior even though they are no longer receiving any external positive rewards.

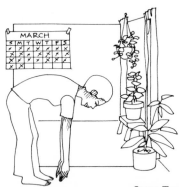

Steps Toward Behavioral Change

This recording continues to help maintain a focus on the new behavior and the changes which have occurred. Thus, a person who engaged in a weight loss program might continue to weigh in on a daily or weekly basis, or a smoker might continue to 'X' off in red on the calendar another day he succeeded in not smoking.

As we mentioned earlier when we discussed Grandma's Law, or the Premack Principle, one of the most effective ways to establish a new behavior is to link it to an already well-established behavior. The well-established habit and the use of continued recording serve as cues to the individual to help maintain his new behavior.

When working with a patient, the use of follow-up appointments or even telephone calls can help ease the transition. It seems that the mere knowledge that someone cares enough to check up on how the person is doing lends some impetus for the individual to follow through. Moreover, it offers an opportunity for you to identify any problems that have developed and possibly work out the kinks. Finally, it helps you discover the kinds of problems your patients have with different intervention strategies—information which helps you design better programs in the future.

When talking with patients during this termination phase, it is important to emphasize that problems, particularly backsliding, often occur, and that this is not evidence of their inability to change or their lack of willpower, but rather the difficulty of change. One of the most common reasons for backsliding is a change of routine by the individual. When a person moves, takes a new job, marries, or even takes a vacation, his routines change and new habits can easily be lost in the shuffle.

Some backsliding is to be expected, but it does not mean that the effort was all for naught. You can emphasize to your patients that when this happens—and for most of us backsliding will—they now know the basic tools and techniques that can be used to help implement change, and they can at any time make use of these on their own and apply them to themselves to reestablish any lost behavior.

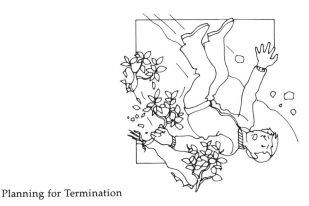

You have shown them a systematic approach that they can readily apply to a variety of problems to help them change what they do.

Perspective

At this point we have covered the six fundamental steps involved in initiating a change program. By participating in the change project we recommend, you will experience the different phases of the program and be aware of both the difficulties and advantages involved in each step. Moreover, from your own experience in managing change, you will become familiar with the difficulties inherent in changing someone's behavior.

In your own practice, you may not have the opportunity, or even find it necessary, to go through each step with every patient who desires change. However, you now possess a basic understanding of the process which occurs when a person tries to alter his behavior. Drawing from this understanding, you should be able to choose the particular sequence of steps or techniques most appropriate to each individual patient.

We do not recommend that you immediately eliminate your present preventive program and substitute our procedures. Rather, it would be best, especially while you are gaining experience with behavior change strategies, to use them to supplement existing procedures.

As with any other procedure or program you employ, remember to approach the patient confidently. Your expectations are always perceived by the patient and will influence whether the patient will be successful in changing his behavior. Aside from the techniques and strategies we have stressed, your enthusiasm and encouragement are the most important factors in helping your patients change their oral habits.

Dentistry, like medicine, has traditionally been disease-oriented. Yet there has always been a recognition that the primary focus of health care should be oriented toward prevention rather than cure. Louis Pasteur said, "When [investigating] a disease, I never think of finding a remedy for it, but instead a means of preventing it."* It was with this goal in mind that this book was conceived.

---

* Quote from the address to the Fraternal Association of Former Students of the École Centrale des Arts et Manufacturers, Paris, May 15, 1884.

Your Practice Project

Fourth Assignment

1. Summarize the results of your monitoring and troubleshooting.
   a. Chart progress on graphs.
   b. Discuss problems that emerged.
   c. Specify changes in intervention plans, objectives, etc., that are needed.

2. Describe specific plans for termination of the project.

Special Management Considerations

The obscure we see eventually; the completely
apparent takes longer.
  E. R. Murrow

7 Treating Special Patients: Children and Elderly

Many health professionals are reluctant to treat children or elderly patients because they fear these patients may present difficult management problems. In some instances, lack of adequate training and experience with children may increase the problem and result in the attitude that treating children is not worth the effort. Similarly, lack of training and experience with the elderly may create problems and uncertainty about whether the elderly are appropriate candidates for dental rehabilitation or preventive care.

Though the principles and strategies we have delineated in the previous chapters can be effective for patients of all ages, we have added this chapter to discuss special considerations for these two populations because practitioners often find they present special problems. Further, the goals of treating special age groups differ from the general treatment goals for the patient population at large.

A number of studies by experts in the field of childhood and pain, such as Forgione and Clark (1974); Kleinknecht, Klepac, and Alexander (1973); Lautch (1971); and Shoben and Borland (1951); show that most people feel that their dental fears began in childhood. Creating positive attitudes toward dental care in children might therefore be the most effective strategy to shape positive attitudes toward dentistry. Early dental experiences must occur with a minimum of physical and psychological trauma. Clinicians as far back as the turn of the century were concerned about the child's fear of dentistry. In 1895, McElroy noted: "Although the operative dentistry may be perfect, the appointment is a failure if the child departs in tears." Just as standard restorative, endodontic, and orthodontic techniques have been modified to treat deciduous dentition, the need to alter patient management has also been recognized. In fact, dental practitioners have long realized that the behavior of the child is the most important factor affecting actual treatment. Without patient cooperation, all dental procedures become difficult; thus the need for effective, humane behavior management of children is obvious.

Considerations for Children

A characteristic of the normal child is that he doesn't act that way very often . . . .

You can learn many things from children. How much patience you have for instance.
   Franklin P. Jones.

Most children seen in the dental office are cooperative and allow the dental care staff to function effectively and efficiently. As a result of long-term water fluoridation, the caries rate has been reduced and children are less likely to need frequent restorative care; without the need for traumatic restorative care children are not as likely to misbehave. Moreover, of the minority who do misbehave, only a few present problems which are serious enough to disrupt treatment. Most misbehavior, such as whining or crying, is merely irritating. When confronted with such behavior, the practitioner can use extinction, or 'time out', very effectively. Though patience and the ability to wait it out are required of the practitioner, the child eventually comes to realize that his behavior will not produce its intended result. Other misbehavior such as passive refusal to 'open wide' or shouts of "I won't" or "I don't want to," or hypermotility—inability to sit still for more than a minute or so—can disrupt efficient treatment. The child who throws a tantrum—screams and flails legs and arms—not only disrupts treatment but endangers patient and staff well-being. Though procedures to manage disruptive and dangerous child behavior exist, measures taken to prevent such extreme behavior from emerging from existing anxiety or fear are well worth the effort. Here we focus on some techniques that you can use when working with children to treat anxiety or fear and prevent problems from developing or becoming unmanageable.

Steps Worth Taking
for Every Child

Establish rapport and communicate effectively. Establishing rapport, one of the foremost objectives when treating children, is not a 'technique' which is applied for a few minutes at the beginning of each appointment. Instead, it is the recognition of each child as a unique individual. Although it is sometimes tempting to act as if children are a different species from adults, current research indicates they are not!

   Your own unique way of responding to adults with whom you are comfortable is also the appropriate way to respond to children in establishing and maintaining rapport. The only difference is that you use simpler concepts and vocabulary with children—without talking

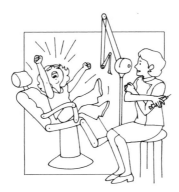

down to them. Children should be talked to at their level of comprehension. That means avoiding baby talk but employing words which have meaning for that patient. Development of your own word substitutes for foreign (to children) dental terminology can be useful; for example, rubber dam becomes rubber raincoat and cotton roll, a tooth pillow. Moreover, the avoidance of scary words such as drill, shot, pain, or the use of euphemisms ("this will feel like a little pinch") will make difficult procedures more acceptable. Practice this as if it were a second language. Everyone in an office should attempt to use the same terminology.

There are many ways to break the ice with children. Questions about their clothing, activities, and pets are commonly used. Whatever the tactic for initiating a conversation, you should plan to use open-ended questions that cannot be responded to in a simple 'yes' or 'no' fashion. For example, do not ask whether the child has a pet—ask him to tell you all about his pets.

Nonverbal communication is also important in establishing rapport. Touching or patting a child's shoulder communicates warmth; smiles convey approval and acceptance. Eye contact is important—when talking to children place yourself at the child's eye level. There is probably some truth in the clinical lore which states that children who avoid eye contact are not ready to cooperate fully.

Administer a parental questionnaire. The parent in the reception room is often a source of information that can help you to better manage the child. Exactly what information should be sought is a function of your individual practice. However, we believe information that will help establish rapport and attune staff to possible behavior problems is extremely valuable. The questions on the following page may be helpful.

1. Does the child have any pets, hobbies, special interests or recent accomplishments?

   Yes ☐   No ☐

   If "yes," please list and/or give kind of pet and names.

2. Does the child have a nickname he enjoys?

   Yes ☐   No ☐

   If "yes," what is it?

3. Name of school _____   Grade _____

4. Other children in family?

   Yes ☐   No ☐

   Please give name, age, and sex of each.

5. Has the child had any unpleasant contact with physicians or dentists?

   Yes ☐   No ☐

   If "yes," please describe.

6. How do you think your child will react to dental treatment?

   Good ☐   Fair ☐   Poor ☐   Don't Know ☐

   Please comment.

7. How would you rate your own anxiety or nervousness at this moment?

   Good ☐   Fair ☐   Poor ☐   Don't Know ☐

8. Has your child had behavior or learning problems at school?

   Yes ☐   No ☐

   Please describe problems.

9. Does your child express concern about aspects of his teeth or mouth, such as a chipped or crooked tooth, decayed tooth, gumboil, etc.?

   Yes ☐   No ☐

   If "yes," please specify.

Studies attempting to identify variables influencing children's behavior in the dental office, summarized nicely in a scholarly review of the literature by Dr. Wright in 1975, have pinpointed three major variables. The pleasantness or unpleasantness of any *previous medical experiences* will affect a child's behavior during his first dental visit. The similarity between dentist and physician is immediately obvious—both are called doctor, wear white coats, and employ receptionists and auxiliaries who dress similarly. Fear, especially in children, is often generalized from one situation to another similar one. *Maternal anxiety* is another variable consistently found to be related to children's behavioral problems. Very anxious mothers have been found to exert a negative influence on children of all ages. The child's *awareness of a dental problem* also creates apprehension which often manifests itself as uncooperative behavior in the dental chair.

Schedule wisely. Initial visits to the dental office are extremely important in that they set the stage for or against dental care for years to come. For preschool children and those with whom you anticipate behavior problems, at first schedule only preclinical visits to familiarize them with the dental environment and personnel. If possible, chart (count) teeth and get the child to respond to directives—for instance, "sit in the chair" or "open your mouth." If the child is very shy or fearful, don't push him.

Scheduling, appointment length, and time of day are important practical considerations. The *schedule* itself may influence cooperative behavior. For instance, there should not be long waiting periods in the reception area. If the child is kept waiting, he may become restless. Experienced pedodontists have also reported that a child who has made positive changes in his behavior should not wait longer than two weeks before the next visit. *Appointment length* is a controversial matter. The trend is now toward longer (30 minutes plus) appointments which allow greater office efficiency. The child is also believed to benefit—he has fewer anesthetic experiences and fewer trips to the dentist's office.

Though researchers have not found that the *time of day* makes a difference, many experienced pedodontists prefer to give young children appointments in the morning and older children appointments in the afternoon. On the other hand, some pedodontists prefer not to see behavior problems first thing in the morning!

Modify the ambience of the office. Though many general practitioners resist making their office child-centered, there are several steps that can be taken to foster a pleasant, positive atmosphere for children. First, the reception room must be inviting. Elaborate redecoration is not necessary. Warm colors, some child-size furniture, and a few toys, games, and books tell the child that this may not be a scary place. Second, smell and taste are important considerations in treating the child. Flavored topical anesthetics, topical fluorides, impression material, and oral premedications are a great help in ensuring receptive children. The opinions of your patients, rather than your own palate, should guide you in reordering supplies. Offensive and unfamiliar odors also must be eliminated. Eliminate or cover the smell of the nasal mask as well as the smell of eugenol, formocresol, and orange oil solutions. Third, visual considerations are important. Most instruments, including syringes, forceps, and bur blocks, should be covered or out of sight—even a glimpse of surgical instruments may induce anxiety and fear-related behavior for some children.

The Guidance-Cooperation Model: A Useful Framework for Interaction with Children. Though a number of specific techniques—Tell-Show-Do, using structured time, the hand-over-mouth procedure—have been discussed in previous chapters, the identification of an overall model of the practitioner-child interaction may be useful in helping you to conceptualize your role and in guiding your selection of specific child management strategies. The following model is derived from the work of two researchers whose contributions not only revitalized their discipline, psychiatry, but also have broader application to all fields of health care delivery. In an article published in 1956, Drs. Szasz and Hollender distinguished three distinct models of doctor-patient relationships: the **active-passive** model, the **guidance cooperation** model, and the **mutual participation** model.

We believe the dental practitioner-child relationship is best characterized as 'guidance-cooperation'. In this model the patient is not completely passive, as is the case in surgery where general anesthesia is required (the active-passive model); neither is the child permitted to participate with the practitioner in decisions concerning the dental procedure to be employed (the mutual participation model). In a treatment situation characterized by guidance-cooperation, the child is expected to look up to and obey the practitioner. This model has its prototype in the relationship of parent and child, and is especially relevant for pedodontics, where the practitioner is in a guiding or helping relationship with a young child who comes for treatment. Recent research by Drs. Wurster, Weinstein, and Domoto, conducted in 1978 at the University of Washington School of Dentistry, has indicated that the use of 'directive guidance'—a straightforward assertive statement of expectation or feedback concerning the child's behavior—led to cooperative child behavior. For example: "If you feel anything, raise your hand like this" (demonstrate), or "Open a little wider, please—Good boy!" On the other hand, permissive behavior, such as saying, "Are you ready for me to begin now?", and coercive behavior, such as threats or scolding, resulted in substantial resistant and uncooperative child behavior.

A number of principles emerge from this model. Two of these, structuring and shaping, have been mentioned in chapter 4.

1. Tell the child the ground rules (before and during treatment). Let the child know what you expect him to do and not to do. For example, "You must do exactly what I tell you to do. All of my helpers always keep their hands on their laps." Structuring time (so the child knows what to expect) may be a useful tactic. For a young child (3 to 7 years), a few minutes may seem an interminable period of time to remain still. An egg timer—one with sand in it is best—is useful to let hypermotile children know how long they must sit still before they will be allowed playtime or stretch time. This is initiated before a procedure. Needless to say, you must live up to the agreement.

   Note: Movement in the dental chair is normal for all preadolescent children and is not itself indicative of a hyperactive child.

2. Praise all cooperative behaviors. You cannot praise or 'stroke' the child too frequently. When the child makes any attempt to respond to a directive, for example, "open wide," praise him to shape his behavior. Most importantly, do not forget to praise him when he is sitting still and cooperating. Too often, we do not pay attention to the child until his behavior causes problems.

3. Keep your cool. To show anger in response to a child's behavior will only make matters worse. If you can ignore irritating but non-interfering behavior such as crying or whining, do so. If you cannot, do not retaliate with coercion.

   We are not saying you should not show your displeasure. A statement like "I get mad (or unhappy, etc.) when you . . . ," when said in a calm voice, is more likely to succeed than coercion or permissiveness.

4. Use voice control. Frequently a sudden change in tone or volume can be used to gain the attention of a child who is not cooperating. What is said is not critical; it is the change of voice that gains the attention of the child. Return to the previous tone or volume as soon as the child begins to respond to your voice change.

5. Allow the child to play a role. Structure choices for the child to make. For example, "Shall we count the top or bottom teeth first?" . . . "Would you like me to help you into the chair or would you like to climb up yourself?" Do not, unless you are willing to abide by his decision, ask the child if he wants to get into the chair or open his mouth.

   Most children want to be as adult as possible and enjoy the role of 'helper'. Helpers hold mirrors, swabs, etc., and receive praise for the good work they do. This is especially useful for preschoolers.

6. Avoid attempting to talk a child into cooperation. Do not give lengthy explanations of why a procedure is needed. Instead, ac-

knowledge the child's feelings, "You don't like taking pictures." You may even follow with a verbal wish that it was not necessary or that it would be more fun to be outside playing. Then firmly request cooperation.

It should also be pointed out that confidence is important in working with children, and that it usually develops from experience. Our research tells us that confident practitioners use more directive guidance and less coercion and permissive behavior when compared to the less confident practitioners. In addition, as you would probably expect, our research indicates that practitioners who are more confident have greater child cooperation; those who are less confident experience more resistant and uncooperative behavior by children.

How to Deal with Parents. Early in this chapter, we noted that highly anxious mothers tend to have uncooperative children. Interestingly, researchers have found that when mothers attempt to reduce their children's anxieties, they paradoxically increase anxiety. Apparently many mothers (and fathers) do not know how to prepare their children for dental visits. One practical approach to this problem involves sending a preappointment letter to parents of new child patients. In a study published in 1973, Drs. Wright, Alpein, and Leake report success with a letter that read like this:

Dear Mrs. _____ :

I am writing you because I am pleased with the interest you are showing in your child's dental health by making an appointment for a dental examination. Children who have their first dental appointment when they are young are likely to have a favorable outlook toward dental care throughout life.

At our first appointment we will examine your child's teeth and gums, and take any necessary X rays. For most children this proves to be an interesting and even pleasant occasion. All of the people on our staff enjoy children and know how to work with them.

Parents play a most important role in getting children started with a good attitude toward dental care, and your cooperation is much appreciated. One of the useful things that you can do is to be completely natural and easygoing when you tell your child about his appointment. This approach will enable him to view his appointment primarily as an opportunity to meet some new people who are interested in him and want to help him to stay healthy.

Good general health depends in large part upon the development of good habits, such as sensible eating and sleeping routines, exercise, recreation, and the like. Dental health also depends upon good habits, including proper tooth-brushing, regular visits for dental care, and avoidance of excessive sweets. We will have a chance to discuss these points further during your child's appointment.

Best wishes, and I look forward to seeing you.

Should you allow the parent in the operatory? Though the experts tend to disagree, we believe the mother or father should be allowed to remain in the operatory (1) if the patient is not highly anxious, and (2) as long as the child behaves. At times, especially with young children, the parent may be helpful in reducing anxiety and increasing cooperation. Such procedures also avoid compounding the effect of traumatic separation. However, it is important to communicate with the parents and give them the ground rules—that is, that you are the expert and they must respond, even if they do not at the moment personally agree with your approach.

The importance of communication cannot be overstressed—the lines of communication must remain open. Special kinds of communication problems exist for both the special age groups discussed in this chapter, although the nature of these problems is quite different for each group. For the child, the dental office may seem like an unfamiliar and threatening environment. The limited ability of both practitioner and child to communicate often characterizes child-practitioner interactions. On the other hand, elderly patients' loss of vision, hearing, and motor skills affects their ability to communicate. Further, many elderly individuals visit the dental office infrequently, if ever—often for emergency services only. For many different reasons, the elderly patient may have a host of negative attitudes. To provide optimal care rapport with either group is especially important, and the communication process itself may set up difficult barriers that need to be circumvented.

Considerations for Elderly Patients

Growing old isn't so bad when you consider the alternative.
  Maurice Chevalier

Giving up is the ultimate tragedy.
  R. J. Donovan

The need for special consideration for the elderly is not always apparent, nonetheless the needs of the elderly are different from those of all other age groups, and treatment goals also differ. One of the most frustrating experiences for dental health care students and practitioners is a patient's failure to accept or respond to optimal treatment. But in treating the elderly, the difficulty lies in the fact that optimal treatment may be clinically, financially, or psychologically impossible. Often, decisions that we as dental health care providers are not totally comfortable with must be reached. Consequently, our role is not always curative; rather, we must help the patient to develop the best possible adaptation given the restrictions of his physiological and environmental circumstances. Some practitioners may feel unprepared or unable to provide care to elderly patients because they do not understand their special needs. And in some cases patients must be treated in unfamiliar nursing homes or institutional settings and, therefore, present additional obstacles.

Who are the elderly? Many people over 65 vehemently disagree with the societal line of demarcation at age 65. Actually, there is no precise chronological point at which old age can be said to have set in. Rather, it is fluid—a series of gradual modifications which begin at an early age. Many variables such as heredity, working conditions, climate, economics, and a host of unknown factors produce conditions recognized as biological old age, although the chronological age may vary.

Certain chronic conditions such as osteoporosis, osteoarthritis, atherosclerosis, and chronic brain syndrome are commonly associated with old age. In addition, there are a number of accidents and diseases which are experienced over the years—the sum total of which cause the health or ill health of the elderly patient. But, it is not wise to think of the elderly as a homogeneous group.

The variation in health and psychological state from individual to individual is no more amazing than such variation in any age group. Moreover, the elderly patient's response to stressful situations, for example, a visit to the dentist or physician, is not a function of either chronological or biological age. Characteristic patterns of responding to stress—like dependency, passive-aggression, hostility, and denial—have developed throughout a lifetime. The problems of aging only serve to intensify and exaggerate existing patterns. On the other hand, it is possible that flexible, competency-related coping patterns are extinguished in continuing unsuccessful interactions with younger individuals, while rigid, stereotyped behavior is at the same time reinforced.

We would like to dispel false stereotypes and present rational guidelines for treatment of the elderly in the dental office. You should keep in mind, however, that our statements are generalizations and do not hold for every elderly patient you encounter. Temper your management by careful observation of each elderly individual in your care.

Dental Needs of the Aged. The oral cavity, like other parts of the body, is not immune to the problems of chronic diseases associated with the aging process. In a scholarly review of geriatric research published in 1967, Drs. Anderson and Anderson indicate that the elderly have the greatest oral health needs of any segment of our population. For example, in 1968 a well-known figure in the field of oral pathology, Dr. Bhaskar, reported an 81% incidence of pathology in elderly institutionalized patients who presented no obvious symptoms and were under "optimal care." Soft tissues revealed 19 types of diseases ranging from innocuous areas of pigmentation to early squamous cell carcinoma.

Oral health is particularly problematic for the elderly edentulous patient. Within a short time of fitting dentures there frequently is deterioration and a tendency for patients to overadapt to change. Dentures are frequently used well beyond their normal life. Many elderly edentulous patients do not seek prosthetic treatment which could enable them to have better mastication and would eliminate the almost universal irritation of denture-bearing tissue. With poor dental health, the elderly patient will tend to select a diet that fails to meet bodily needs, consuming food low in proteins and high in carbohydrates and fats.

Though some of these problems are a result of the aging process itself, others are related primarily to attitudes toward the consequences of aging and resultant neglect. Older persons tend to react passively to the effects of aging on external body features and appearance, and they are less likely than younger individuals to be concerned about their appearance. Older persons are also more likely to believe all sorts of disability, illness, and pain are an unavoidable part of aging. Consequently, they may have a fatalistic attitude toward their health and are less likely to take steps to guard their physical well-being. In general, concern with prevention of disease seems to decline with age. Dental visits and home care activities are definitely affected. In their report of the proceedings of the National Conference of Dentistry and Geriatrics at Harvard, 1972, Drs. Fishman and Bikofsky indicated that although financial restrictions are often the reason for this decline in care, many elderly people do not take advantage of free care even when it is offered.

Though there is a correlation between aging and dental disease, the relationship is not necessarily causal. Dental educators and researchers are now attempting to foster a rehabilitative-preventive approach to the oral problems of the aged. These professionals catalogue problems of diseased and missing teeth, ill-fitting dentures or partial dentures, soft tissue diseases, and bone deterioration as amenable to rehabilitation, if not prevention. Moreover, this approach addresses the consequences of poor oral health in the elderly: poor diet leading to malnutrition, pain, infection, even impaired social functioning, all problems that are treatable or preventable.

But precisely such attitudes as those mentioned above that are common among the elderly can be barriers to the success of dental care. Among the elderly who accept illness as inevitable, many are not interested in what they perceive to be 'superficial aspects' of their bodies, and among professionals there are some who hold the same view, or are simply not interested in treating the aged. Providing preventive care to elderly patients is challenging; it is often difficult to motivate them to seek dental care or to prevent problems that they do not believe to be severely handicapping.

We would now like to suggest some considerations that, though not unique to the elderly, are especially important to keep in mind when working with this population.

Steps Worth Taking for Elderly Patients

Establish rapport. Time invested in establishing rapport with older patients is not wasted. You should appear unhurried and take time to pass the time of day' with the patient. A general suspicion of professionals by many elderly patients warrants your conveying a personal interest in them. Try to have as much closeness in face-to-face communication as is comfortable. Remember, their visual and auditory losses require much closer interpersonal distances. Avoid physical barriers—sit next to the patient, not behind a desk. Physical contact is also reassuring.

Gradually introduce into the conversation your questions about previous dental care—they may provoke revealing answers. Perhaps the patient is worried about cost or discomfort. Or perhaps he does not really want dental care and came only at the insistence of a relative or friend. Patients' answers to questions about loss of teeth and the wearing of dentures are also helpful in planning future treatment.

Treat elderly patients with dignity. Care should be taken not to threaten the elderly individual's self-esteem, as it is important for survival. In addition, many elderly people are sensitive to their loss of status and esteem; therefore, it is extremely important to treat them with dignity and courtesy. Remember that through death of

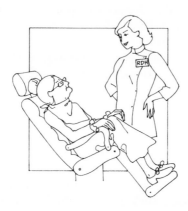

Special Management Considerations

loved ones, loss of work role and financial security, and reduction of physical abilities, many elderly persons have lost their own sense of competence and independence. Involve the patient in treatment planning. When ready to consult with the patient, move from the operatory to the office. Such special attention reduces tension and supports a positive self-image. Often because their self-image has become less positive, elderly patients do not seek health care.

Some practitioners find that write-ups of diagnosis and treatment plans are useful. Whether or not you use such a plan, you should encourage the elderly patient not to make an immediate decision, especially if feelings about the treatment plan appear uncertain. The patient should have time to decide or seek the opinion of other professionals. When, for example, the patient decides to have dentures, it is helpful to involve him in the selection of teeth. This will result in fewer complaints, corrective work, and rejections.

Expect active participation. Request that your elderly patients maintain their own oral hygiene, as you would do with other patients. Many practitioners may inadvertently discourage the self-maintaining behaviors of the elderly by unburdening them of responsibilities for their own self-maintenance. Encourage them to strive for some level of competence and control over their lives. When treated as deficient, most patients will react by meeting your low expectations. Self-fulfilling prophecies occur at all ages.

From the studies of psychologists Kastenbaum (1968); Libb and Clements (1969); and Hoyer and associates (1975); it is noted that behavior change techniques have been applied to a variety of problematic behavior patterns of elderly persons, although a few minor adjustments may be necessary. There is some evidence that the elderly need more encouragement than those who are younger. High ratios of reinforcement of effort are also encouraged, as is strong support or reinforcement from those in the home environment. Objectives should be relatively short-term and uncomplicated, as long-range, complex plans are especially likely to have a negative influence on the decisions and behavior of many elderly people.

Assess psychological factors. Prior to extensive and expensive dental work, evaluation of the patient's personal values regarding the importance of oral health, his more general approach to life, and his relationship to you are critical. These are important factors in his satisfaction with your work and may relate to how well the patient will maintain a prosthetic appliance or program of oral hygiene. Dr. Siefert, studying dental care satisfaction and the geriatric patient, demonstrated in a study published in 1972 that a positive approach to life and people, as opposed to a critical or disturbed approach, is conducive to satisfaction with dental care, as is perception of the practitioner as helpful and kind. Moreover, the level of patient satisfaction could not be correlated with either intelligence (beyond the ability to comprehend what is said) or previous dental experience. The practitioner's best source of data for assessing these factors is the patient's verbal and non-verbal behavior during his interaction with the staff in the dental setting.

Go slowly. Though aging does not necessarily result in deterioration of mental abilities, the elderly seem to need more time to absorb information or make decisions. Their comprehension is as great as that of younger individuals, but they tend to be cautious. They want to be accurate. These concerns prevent immediate or rapid reaction. The rate at which you present material is of great importance. It is wise to give instructions slowly and clearly—written instructions are an effective follow-up to verbal direction. Careful arrangement of material is also important—the less complex the better. When attempting to learn new skills, for example, proper brushing or flossing, everyone's performance usually begins at a low level and increases with practice. The elderly need more repetitions and pauses during practice in order to reach the same standards as those reached by younger people.

We have nothing to fear but fear itself.
 F.D.R.

8 Anxiety, Fear, Phobias, and Pain

Why We Included This Chapter

After much thought, we have included a last chapter to focus on the subject of fear and anxiety. Although fear and anxiety do not directly relate to behavior change of oral health care habits, they are without question major problems with which every dental professional must cope. For anxiety and fear may significantly interfere with a successful attempt at any behavior change.

Beyond presenting immediate problems in the operatory, we believe anxiety and fear may explain why some patients have management problems—that is, they "know how but don't do." For example, some patients report they have put off making dental appointments for fear of finding something wrong with their teeth. We are all familiar with the patient who repeatedly cancels appointments, or the patient who waits "until it hurts" before scheduling an appointment. We believe that the dental professional can do much to prevent and relieve patient anxieties and fears—first, by teaching the patient how to establish and maintain adequate home care skills so that he learns that he has no cause to worry; and second, in conjunction with some basic techniques that help people cope with stressful situations, by familiarizing the patient with dental procedures to reduce the 'fear of the unknown' and 'feelings of helplessness'.

A caution: All the techniques discussed in this chapter have been found effective in the dental setting; however, just like any other procedure, they are difficult to learn by simply reading about them. For some of you, the techniques we discuss will seem familiar and similar to what you already do. For others, this material may be totally new. This chapter makes no attempt to be a comprehensive guide to the use of these techniques. We suggest you proceed cautiously in adapting these procedures, applying those techniques which seem to fit most comfortably with your own management style. Attempting new procedures under the watchful eyes of an expert may also prove valuable.

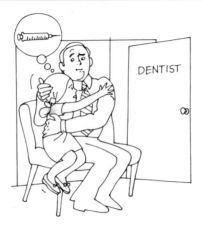

Fear and Anxiety
What Are They

Most patients experience some degree of anxiety, fear, or pain when visiting the dental office. When dental care was provided almost entirely by dentists who were for the most part repairmen and patients were perceived as conveyors of diseased dentition, these issues were not of much concern. Today, with the emphasis upon prevention and increasing recognition of patient rights, it is critical for all dental health care providers to understand how anxiety, fear, and pain affect the course of dental treatment.

The problems confronting the dental practitioner are, in some ways, unique. Bertram Levin, a highly respected medical educator, made an often quoted observation: "Our first patient is our silent uncomplaining cadaver. Some among us," he added, "think this is the model of what the proper patient ought to be—silent, uncomplaining, endlessly tolerant and unperturbed by your mistakes! The dentist, however, is the surgeon who does not have a cadaver or a totally anesthetized patient to work with, and must combine technical competence with chairside manner that will sustain the patient through the experience."

Before reviewing specific techniques you can use as part of your chairside manner' to help the patient (and you) cope with fear, anxiety, and pain, we need to examine (1) what these terms actually mean, and (2) how such feelings originate.

Anxiety may best be thought of as a *general* state of nervousness. It is usually very difficult for the patient to define, except in very broad terms, what it is he is anxious about. The origin of anxiety appears most often to originate from either (1) some vague past remembrance of unpleasant situations, or (2) learning from what peers, relatives, and the media say or do, without ever actually experiencing a specific anxiety-producing event. That is, anxiety may be the result of others modeling attitudes and behavior which come to influence the patient's own opinions and feelings.

Fear may be thought of as anxiety about a specific identifiable situation, event, or person, or, to use the psychological term, stimulus. The stimulus may be something very specific, such as injection needles, or a more general class of events—such as going to a dental appointment. Fear most frequently originates from some direct negative experience, although it is not unusual to find a person fearful solely as a result of peer or parental modeling. As a result of such modeling, children are frequently highly fearful at their first nontreatment appointment.

A **phobia** may be defined as fear that is clearly *irrational*, an over-response to a specific situation or stimulus much greater than is warranted. For example, a person with a snake phobia might burst into hysterical screaming upon seeing a small garden snake in a cage. A phobic exhibits extreme fear and an inability to discuss rationally the object of the phobia. Even a painful toothache may not be enough to bring a true phobic into the dental office. It should be pointed out, however, dental care practitioners seldom meet dental phobics.

And, finally, **pain.** At first glance, pain is seemingly easy to identify—in reality it is a very elusive concept. Pain is defined as a *subjective* feeling of extreme discomfort. It is classified into two basic types: (1) acute, such as from an injection; and (2) chronic, for example, myofacial pain.

The Origins of Fears Related to Dental Care

Having briefly examined the terms and their relationship to one another, let's focus in more detail on the public's perception of dental care. What are the major sources of fear in the dental environment? In a survey of dental fears reported in 1973, Drs. Kleinknecht, Klepac and Alexander found the highest fear ratings were given to the sight of the syringe and sensation of the injection. The next most fear-producing stimuli were the sight, sound, and feeling of the drill—results no experienced clinician would find surprising.

In conducting their study, Kleinknecht and his colleagues asked 487 patients about their perceptions of the causes of their fears. The most commonly offered cause was the negative influence of others. Almost 17% of the participants mentioned that stories told by friends and relatives, television, cartoons, and other media had given them expectations of being traumatized by dental treatment. The second most frequently mentioned category (13.5%) was previous painful dental work. The third most frequent category was perceived errors (8.3%) on the part of the practitioner. The fourth category was poor management (6.8%).

Included in this last category of poor management were threats to patients if they did not cooperate, refusal to use an anesthetic when requested, and starting dental work before the anesthetic took effect. Although the validity of the patient viewpoints may not be totally accurate, what is important is that the participants in the study perceived their viewpoints as true, and their perceptions led to fear.

Prevalence of Dental Fears

How common is fear of dental care in the general population? In a national survey of dental health conducted in 1958 by two prominent sociological researchers, Friedson and Feldman, it was found that of the 51% of the population who reported not seeing a dentist regularly, 9% gave fear as the primary reason. In another sociological study, Dr. Crocket reported in 1965 that 5% to 6% of the general population and as high as 16% of school-aged children avoided dental care because of fear. In 1976 Drs. Kleinknecht and Bernstein, in a survey of fearful dental patients, found that 80% of the individuals considering themselves highly fearful had put off making dental appointments, and 50% had cancelled existing appointments. Of those individuals who considered themselves to have a moderate or low amount of fear, only 2.6% had put off making dental appointments. None of the low-fear group had ever cancelled appointments.

The research of Kleinknecht and Bernstein also revealed that women tend to rate themselves more fearful than men. However, in their studies conducted about the frequency of dental visits in the general population, a significantly greater percentage of females than males went to the dentist regularly. It is difficult to draw any definite conclusions from these data. It may be that women are simply more willing to admit their fears than are men. There may be any number of reasons why more females than males see the dentist regularly. It may be that it is easier for more women than men to find time, as a smaller percentage work full time. It may be that since mothers are often the parent responsible for their children's health care, they make appointments for themselves as well as for their children when they are taken to the dental office. Or, it may be that societal pressure to maintain physical attractiveness is greater for females.

Finally, one last statistic: When Drs. Friedson and Feldman (1958) asked whether "a person should make a practice of seeing the dentist regularly, every six months or a year, even when his teeth are all right, or is it not worth the trouble unless there is some discomfort," 88% of the respondents answered that regular visits were a good idea. However, only 68% of them had actually been to the dentist in the past twelve months. Once again, it is evident that knowing what you should do, or what is good for you, does not necessarily lead to positive action.

The Fear Process

Having looked at the prevalence of fear in the general population, let's focus on the process of how an individual becomes fearful. When you ask people about their fears, a response that is not uncommon is, "I just have these feelings," or "I can't control them," which all somehow implies that they come from outside the person.

It is important to remember, as we mentioned in chapter 3, that behavior—which includes fears, anxieties, phobias, and, to a large extent, pain—is learned. Fear, anxiety, and phobias are behavioral and psychological responses to stress. Any time an individual is required to cope with, or adapt to, environmental circumstances, stress is produced. Drs. Thomas H. Holmes and Richard Rahe, psychiatrists at the University of Washington, devised a scale of events as shown on the next page. They found that change, whether for good or bad, causes stress and leaves us more susceptible to disease. Even events that we find positive, such as graduation, promotions, Christmas, or an eagerly awaited vacation, produce stress.

How we cope with fear, anxiety, pain, or other stressors is also learned. The well-known behavioral psychologist, Bernstein, in a recent study reports findings which do not support the typical cultural stereotypes. He found that, "while personally communicated anecdotes, television, and films support (and even produce) the expectation that virtually everyone is afraid of dentists, dentists report that only 5% to 16% of their patients display negative emotional reactions of a magnitude sufficient to regularly interfere with treatment procedures." The number of patients who on occasion experience fear and thus become management problems no doubt increase the percentages reported by Bernstein. However, the point is that most of us, even though we experience fear, have learned how to control our fear and anxiety in a socially acceptable way. Those individuals who are less successful at coping, like "Chicken Little," focus on catastrophizing ideas, which in turn may heighten anxiety. In addition, it should be noted that how much pain a patient feels and/or reports to others is dependent to a large extent upon the specific coping skills that he has developed.

Past experiences with pain and exposure to how 'significant others' (parents, spouses, and peers) handle pain are extremely influential. We have learned that cultural patterning and training shape and reinforce pain-related behavior. For example, Eskimos have been reported to respond to pain with laughter. The consistency and intensity of social reinforcement affects an individual's perception of the severity, and his display of pain. Athletes involved in contact sports for a number of years learn to ignore pain and not talk about it, as they have had repeated exposure to the negative responses of their fellow players to displays of pain.

Life Event*	Scale of Impact
Death of spouse	100
Divorce	73
Personal injury or illness	53
Marriage	50
Fired at work	47
Change in health of family member	44
Pregnancy	40
Change in financial state	38
Change in responsibilities at work	29
Outstanding personal achievement	28
Change in living conditions	25
Change of personal habits	24
Change in work hours or conditions	20
Change in residence	20
Change in social activities	18
Change in eating habits	15
Vacation	13
Christmas	12
Minor violations of the law	11

* From: Holmes, T.H. and Rahe, R.H. The social adjustment rating scale. J. Psychosm. Res., 11:213, 1967—by permission of Pergamon Press, Ltd., New York.

Fear Prevention and Fear Reduction

It is easy to make a conceptual distinction between procedures geared toward preventing fear acquisition on the one hand, and techniques for reducing already-acquired fear on the other. Prevention seems reducible to 'don't hurt the patient'. It seems logical that if stimuli—drills, injections, and the like—in the dental office are not repeatedly paired with intense pain, fear should not develop. However, such a view represents only a half-truth.

There is no doubt that first-hand experiences with pain in the unique and rich set of stimuli which comprise the dental office play a

Special Management Considerations

role in the acquisition of some of the fears associated with dental care. Dr. Lautch reported in 1971, for example, that only 10 of 34 fearless dental patients reported one traumatic painful experience with dental work, and only one reported two such experiences. In contrast, all 34 fearful patients reported one traumatic experience, and 30 of them reported two or more. (The four fearful subjects who reported only one painful experience never returned to the dentist's office for a second appointment.) When considered with other similar self reports (Kleinknecht, Klepac, and Alexander, 1973) and laboratory studies of fear and avoidance, pain cannot be denied as a factor contributing to the origins of dental fear in patients.

However, practicing dentists often see a number of cases where children on their first visit to a dentist are already highly fearful (Papermaster, 1971). Data presented by other researchers (Shoben and Borland, 1954) also suggest that generalization from prior experiences with physicians, modeling of fearful behavior by others, and vicarious learning may often render a child fearful prior to his first encounter with dental care.

Although eliminating pain from a child's early interactions with dental practitioners is desirable, it cannot be expected to eliminate all, nor perhaps most fear of dental care. Prevention of dental fear may, in most cases, translate into the reduction of already acquired fear. The dental literature suggests little difference between techniques described as "preventive" and those described as "therapeutic." Making distinctions between preventing fear and treating acquired fear is not difficult semantically. Behaviorally, in the operatory, it's a formidable, if not impossible task.

Recognizing the Basic Signs of Anxiety. Each of us in dental health care soon begins to recognize signs that indicate a patient is nervous—whether we are able to verbalize them or not. Some of the basic signs of fear and anxiety follow.

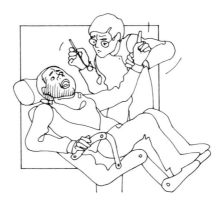

Verbal indicators. These include: talking too much or too rapidly—jumping rapidly from subject to subject; making inappropriate jokes; talking too little, such as answering in one word responses; talking inappropriately loud; or talking too quietly. In reading this list, the question that comes immediately to mind is, what do we mean by talking "too loud" or "talking inappropriately"? There is no one standard against which the behavior of every individual can be compared. In this respect, interpreting what you observe is an art as well as a skill.

Behavioral indicators. The range of behavioral signs seems almost limitless. Some of the more common include nervous laughter or smiles when there is no apparent cause; short, clipped endings to words; the voice cracking; trembling hands; rubbing hands together continually; gripping the chair tightly with both hands; continual cancelled or broken appointments; and consistent lateness to appointments.

Physiological indicators. The physiological responses to stress are less observable, but there are several signs that can be observed: dilated eyes; white knuckles; perspiration on hands, forehead, and above the lip; redness in the neck below the ear; uneven breathing; or a dry mouth.

Many of us intuitively learn to recognize some of these signs. None of them is a foolproof indicator (the patient may have just run two blocks to your office), but they can serve as a set of cues to help you determine how the patient is feeling.

Once you have tentatively identified signs of anxiety in your patient, the next fundamental step is to check out your perceptions or hunches. Communication is the key to help you determine whether the patient is in fact anxious, and if so what course of action you wish to take. Communication is also the most fundamental method you have of helping a patient cope with fear and anxiety.

Taking time to obtain an accurate picture of the patient and his particular situation is crucial. For example, many practitioners find children fearful of the dental appointment even though they may have had little or no previous experience. Discussion with the mother or child may reveal that the parent or a sibling has set the stage by relating horror stories.

" . . . they lay you back in this chair and bring out a tray full of these horrible tools, great big pliers, long sharp things they stick in your mouth, and then they give you a shot with a huge needle!"

It is not difficult to see why many of us are afraid before we even go to the dental office. As we noted, discussion with the parent may help you find out how the child normally deals with stress, and what kind of cues he gives before acting disruptively. Also, the use of a preappointment letter explaining normal procedures and asking a few questions regarding past medical and dental experiences may provide potential areas to discuss with the patient.

You should always be aware that your voice has a very important influence on how the patient perceives the event taking place. Fearful patients tend to pay special attention to incongruities between inflection and tone and the content of your message. Having an opportunity to record yourself on videotape, or simply setting up an audio cassette recorder in the clinic and listening to your interactions with a patient can provide you with valuable information and feedback.

Another part of effective communication is encouraging the patient to verbalize or ventilate his feelings. It helps the patient to relieve anxiety and fear if he is encouraged to express his feelings and knows that they are understood, or that others also have such feelings. Your verbal recognition or acknowledgment of anxiety and other feelings can help bring the issues out into the open. For example, statements such as "I bet that you'd really rather be somewhere else," or acknowledgment that "It isn't all that pleasant to be here," help show your awareness of the patient's thoughts and feelings. At other times you may wish to inquire directly about how the patient is feeling, "Are you feeling a little nervous about the appointment today?"

Checking out what you observe is a low-risk strategy which encourages the patient to open up and explain in his own words how the experience is affecting him. For example, "You seem to be sweating," or "You seem to be grasping the chair very tightly." Compare this approach to one where you label or tell the patient what he is feeling, such as "You are really very anxious, aren't you?"

Studies have repeatedly confirmed that, when under stress, people prefer to be with others and they especially like to relate to a confident figure of authority. Recognizing patient anxiety, encouraging the patient to verbalize, and making observational statements are all part of utilizing people's need for affiliation and understanding.

Clearly establishing two-way communication between you and the patient is a very effective way of helping the patient cope with his anxieties and fears. Many patients do not feel they have the right to ask questions about treatment or make comments to the practitioner. To help initiate or ensure two-way communication, the dental health professional must make it clear to the patient that such communication is expected. A simple but frequently used method is to tell the patient to raise his hand when a procedure begins to hurt, or when a pause is desired. Another is simply telling the patient that it is O.K. to ask questions, or to ask for rest periods. Each of these methods helps eliminate feelings that the patient is helpless or at the mercy of the practitioner, or that "he never tells me anything."

Using Drugs to Reduce Anxiety

The second most widely used method of helping patients cope with fear and anxiety is drugs. Quick, easy, and often effective, they are tempting to use, but also subject to misuse and abuse. Effective in reducing mild or moderate anxiety, drugs can be dramatically counterproductive with patients who seemingly need them the most—the severely anxious. In a lecture presented in 1977 to the dental students at the University of Washington, Dr. Samuel F. Dworkin, a distinguished pain researcher with degrees in psychology and dentistry, addressed the question of drugs in reducing anxiety as follows.

Paradoxically, it often turns out that the most anxious patients are the most resistant to analgesic and sedative drugs that we want to use for control of anxiety. Patients highly anxious about general things like loss of control, fear of the unknown, and loss of support, view Valium, Demerol, and IVs equally as threatening as operatory procedures. And so, it very often turns out that the very pharmaceutical methods you use for pain control and sedation are not effective in the people who seem to need them the most. In children, there is a phenomenon known as barbiturate reversal. When you give short-acting barbiturates to children, they can become physically impossible to control. Providing dental care is then impossible even in an emergency situation where you have to do some dental work.

   If you try to use audio-analgesic techniques—putting on headphones and music or static for very anxious people—patients rip them off because they have no room in their heads to deal with anything but controlling their own anxieties. It is not the dentistry that is the obnoxious agent for them, it is the internal experience of their own anxieties. Anxiety is also the biggest compounder of pain response.

   We strongly encourage systematic desensitization procedures, relaxation techniques, and other behavior modification techniques that are very effective, and work well. However, to be effective, such techniques must come out of the unique relationship you develop with your patient. As with any technique, the patient must perceive that you care about helping him with the problem. He must come to trust you, and what you are trying to do. Pharmaceuticals are not a panacea—if you use them at all, you should limit yourself to a few drugs so that you can maximize your experience with these agents and master their use. And, pharmaceuticals are not a substitute for a good practitioner-patient relationship.

Other Approaches
to Reducing Anxiety

Desensitizing. A procedure useful in reducing the anxiety of both the adult and young patient is called **desensitizing.** For the child who has never received dental treatment, we recommend that the first appointment serve to desensitize or slowly and carefully introduce the

Special Management Considerations

child to the dental environment. The child should be reinforced for all cooperating behavior and should receive some tangible reinforcement at the end of the visit. At the next visit the experienced clinician will be able to judge whether the child is ready for a full session of operative dentistry or if a more gradual, step-by-step introduction to treatment is required. A variation of this procedure is also possible with anxious adults.

The popular **Tell-Show-Do** method, formalized into a technique by noted pedodontist Dr. Addelston (1959), is extremely effective with children who are not severely anxious. It is based upon the principles of prompting, shaping, and reinforcement. For example, once the child is settled in the chair you might say:

"Now I am going to take about five minutes and count your teeth." (This is the 'Tell', a prompt.)

"This is the mirror that will help me see your teeth and the counter that will help me touch and count each tooth." (This is the 'Show', which involves shaping.)

"Now open wide. . . . Very good, I see you have one, two, three teeth. Now let's look at the bottom teeth." (This is the 'Do'. Social reinforcement should immediately follow appropriate behavior.)

Experts say that it is important to use Tell-Show-Do at each step of a procedure so that the child becomes familiar with the dental environment and the appointment is broken up into brief time periods. Structuring events to have a definite beginning and end is easier for the young child to accept than one long unbroken stretch of time in which there is no end in sight. With older, more experienced children or adults, the Tell-Show-Do method can cover several procedural steps at a time.

Control. Most people are to some degree afraid of, or bothered by, feelings of helplessness or loss of control during the dental appointment. Determining the amount of control the patient wants over the dental situation may be critical.

There are three basic types of control. The most obvious is **behavioral control**—the ability to actually control what happens. The opportunity for this type of control for the patient is, of course, limited. However, when the patient is able to raise his hand to stop the drilling, request that the chair be readjusted, or ask for a brief rest period, he is exercising behavioral control of the situation.

Decisional control is having and exercising choices of what will happen, or in what order or when events will occur. Examples include deciding in advance how long the appointment will be, or what work will be accomplished first. Asking the child if he wants to get into the chair from the left or right side, or if he wants his bottom or top teeth checked first, is another example.

Third, **cognitive control** relates to obtaining sufficient information to be able to understand what is going on. Some patients, for example, report discomfort and feelings of helplessness when they have had their glasses removed by the dentist, for they can no longer observe what is going on. Similarly, some patients prefer to observe procedures through the reflection of the clinician's glasses, or through a hand mirror. The Tell-Show-Do technique is a particularly effective procedure to use with children. With adults it might be thought of as familiarization with office equipment and explanation of dental procedures, but it serves a similar function, just like a preappointment letter or a pretreatment appointment, of increasing a patient's cognitive control.

How much information should you try to give the patient? This, too, differs for each individual. Interestingly, studies have shown that severely anxious patients have their anxiety reduced when they receive either a short 'off the cuff' or a long, carefully prepared interview outlining the situation, the operatory procedure, and possible consequences. On the other hand, the anxiety of mildly anxious patients tends to increase following a short interview, and decreases only after a longer, more supportive interview—supporting the old saw that sometimes a little knowledge can be a dangerous thing.

Each individual's need and desire for control in a stressful situation differs. The wish for personal control becomes for most of us a deep-seated desire. However, there appears to be a small, but significant number of people who seem to prefer to relinquish control in a stress-producing situation and rely upon the 'expert'.

How should the practitioner handle individuals who prefer to relinquish control? From your first contact with the patient, as you are beginning to establish communication and rapport, you need to begin assessing the patient's desire for information and control over the treatment process. You can make it clear, for example, that you are receptive to questions, and that there are options available from which the patient can choose—for example, length of appointment times, the order in which the work might be done, how extensive it might be, frequency of appointments—or the patient can decide to leave it all to your best judgment.

For instance, time structuring can be used to let the patient know what can be expected during the appointment. Some individuals feel most comfortable "getting it all over as fast as possible," while others appreciate having prearranged breaks to get up and stretch, or ten minutes in the play room.

Modeling, a strategy to help patients learn new behavior, can also be employed to provide information or cognitive control to patients and help set the stage for cooperative behavior from children and fearful adults. As the anxious or fearful adult or child watches

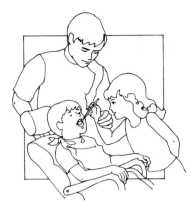

another patient, he not only sees what he can expect, but also observes someone else coping adequately with the situation.

The most critical factor determining the effectiveness of the modeling procedure is that the person perceives the model as fundamentally similar to himself. In other words, a 7-year-old boy watching a 13-year-old girl would have little effect. It is also helpful if the model is perceived as somewhat fearful, but able to overcome his fears and cope adequately. If a model is perceived to be confident and masterful, he is less likely to influence the observer—"He may not be afraid, but I am."

Many practitioners have long used modeling strategies by letting the younger child watch 'big sister' through the appointment if they perceive a positive relationship between a confident sibling and the fearful child. A simple variation of the same strategy involves scheduling an unrelated fearful child to watch another child patient during his appointment.

A more complex use of this strategy involving both the Tell-Show-Do technique and modeling, but which can be successfully used by the practitioner, was described in 1971 by pedodontist Dr. Papermaster.

A 'leader' child, who has had dental work done previously, is seated in the dental chair. One of the new patients is asked to assist in making the dental examination. He is given the mouth mirror and [a blunted] explorer. . . . Assist the child by holding his hand as he examines the teeth with the mouth mirror, checking the cavities and the fillings. He is then given the handpiece and is guided while one or two of the anterior teeth are polished with a rubber cup. He is given a pair of tweezers holding a piece of cotton, and is asked to wipe off any particles on the teeth. The patient who has helped in the examination is then placed in the chair and another youngster is asked to help in the examination, and so on until all the children have been examined. Fillings are done for those who have previously visited the office and the children are dismissed. After one or two Saturday morning appointments, these children can be taken care of at any time during the week in the same manner as any adult.

Anxiety, Fear, Phobias, and Pain

Relaxation. Research studies have shown that a person cannot be both relaxed and tense simultaneously. That is, one cannot be relaxed physically and be preoccupied with anxious thoughts, or be physically tense and be mentally calm. There can be no separation of mind and body.

The relaxation procedure we will discuss is the use of **deep breathing.** Like all the procedures in this chapter, this one can most effectively be mastered by watching and learning from an experienced professional. One characteristic of many anxious individuals, particularly children, is shallow and rapid breathing. In advanced stages of anxiety the patient is literally gasping for air, almost as if he is drowning—and in a sense he is, from his own fear. Once you notice the patient's breathing becoming irregular or increasingly rapid and shallow, there is a simple and remarkably effective breathing exercise to help calm and relax the patient, as well as yourself. This procedure can be used whether the patient is breathing rapidly or at a more normal rate. The following is an example of how it can be used.

With a young child, one might begin by saying, "Before we begin, I'd like to play a game with you. Let's practice holding our breath together, O.K.? Let's take a practice breath first. One, two, three— go." Hold only a few moments and slowly exhale. Praise the child for doing so well and start again—each time holding your breath a little longer. Your purpose is to help the patient get more air and help bring his breathing under control. Then you can talk to the child about slow, deep breathing. "You know what I do when I get afraid? When my heart starts beating real fast and I get afraid, I start breathing like this." Demonstrate by inhaling slowly and deeply, holding for a moment, slowly exhaling, and repeat. Ask the child to join you.

The use of controlled breathing to help reduce anxiety can also be used successfully with adults. Openly acknowledge what you want to do and why. You might begin like this. "I notice you are breathing rapidly. . . . What are you feeling right now?" The patient may or may not verbally acknowledge his rapid breathing or anxiety to you. You can still proceed, however. You might continue by saying something like this, "Whenever I have to do something scary like talk in front of a large group, or when I get to feeling tense before a tennis match or before I take a dive off the high board, it really helps me to take a few deep breaths to relax myself. I'd like to try that with you, O.K.? On the count of three, let's start . . . one, two, three."

Once you and the patient have repeated this several times and his breathing has become more normal, explain that if a person can keep a rich supply of oxygen in his lungs, it helps him to remain more relaxed. You can tell him that you want him to actively practice this procedure during the treatment sessions. Encourage and actively count for him: "In . . . now hold . . . hold . . . exhale."

Focusing on his breathing helps keep the patient physically calm and distracts his attention from thinking about the pain he might suffer.

Cognitive Strategies.*

"The world is such-and-such and so-and-so only because we tell ourselves that that is the way it is. . . . You talk to yourself. . . . You're not unique at that. Every one of us does that. We carry on an internal dialog. . . . We maintain our world with our internal talk."
  C. Castaneda

Modifying **cognitions** is another general strategy. Our cognitions take the form of self-talk, images, and thoughts. These are learned behaviors and undergo constant change. However, sometimes the changes are slow and we find the same self-talk, images, and thoughts repeated over and over until they become automatic and easily triggered by particular events or stimuli.

This is often the case with patients who exhibit stress in the operatory. Early in their dental experience they may have encountered fear or pain. Their interpretation of those experiences may lead to self-talk such as:

"Oh, oh! Look at the instruments! I wonder what tooth he is going to work on? I really get tense when I'm here. I'll hate this but guess there is nothing I can do about it now. I'll just have to let it happen, but it's going to hurt for sure. My body is really tense. I hate coming here."

As the patient reacts to his interpretation of cues—in this case a restorative tray—his body tenses and he becomes anxious. The end result is a fearful, tense patient whose self-talk habits make it less likely he will cope effectively.

Such cognitions take place daily in dental operatories. They often occur as descriptive self-statements—that is, we subvocally describe and interpret our experiences to ourselves. These subvocalizations are our internal reality and in part determine our responses to the outside environment. One of the simplest and most frequently used techniques to control negative cognitions is **attention diversion**.

Attention Diversion. Clinicians have traditionally employed the technique of diverting the attention of the patient to facilitate management. Talking to Larry about his favorite animal while the rubber dam is being placed is an example of this technique. Thus, it is not surprising to note that researchers have determined that diverting the attention of subjects precipitates changes in their perceptions of

---

* This section was written by Gay Davis, M.S.W., University of Washington.

stress and pain. Changes in their responses to stress and the increased degree of tolerance for pain followed.

Research by psychologists J. Horan and J. Dellinger suggests that the nature of the distraction may be important. Subjects who simply count backwards from 100 have no better pain tolerance than those who do nothing; however, those who are distracted by pleasant images endure painful stimulation for longer periods of time.

The airline industry has refined distraction techniques to near perfection. Attractive and attentive personnel, alcohol available at low cost, hot meals, multichannel stereo music, movies, and magazines available for reading are all part of a successful technique which prevents travelers from ruminating about being encased in an aluminum and plastic tube 35,000 feet above the surface of the earth. The professional pickpocket is another testimonial to the slickness of the attention-diversion approach, as the 'mark' seldom realizes that his valuables are gone until long after the thief has disappeared.

Some of the diversion techniques utilized in the dental setting include decorating offices with nontraditional decor and using space to eliminate sights, sounds, and smells traditionally associated with 'doctors' offices'. Music, scenic views, and artwork may act as distracting agents. Patients may sometimes be asked to play an active role in this diversion process. Advising anxious patients to divert their own attention by fantasizing or focusing on a pleasant experience is helpful. Asking patients to concentrate on solving a math problem or riddle during the moment of injection is another example of diversion.

For a majority of patients, information plus some use of distracting techniques often work well together. As mentioned earlier, however, for those patients who have a high fear of loss of control, distraction techniques may actually even be counterproductive. They don't want to be distracted, as their concern is too great. For these patients other stress-reducing techniques should be utilized, especially those giving the patient more control over himself and, when possible, the dental setting and procedure. Another more complex technique involves attempting to modify and change patient cognition (what the patient actually thinks and feels).

Those who experience stressors such as fear and anxiety may be telling themselves things which are quite different from and less calming than the self-talk of those who do not experience such fear and anxiety. Worrying thoughts and catastrophizing self-talk and images may play a major role in the way patients respond in the operatory.

Changing and Modifying Cognitions. Helping the patient control and change these kinds of cognitive behavior is another way to facilitate the effective delivery of dental care. Counterproductive cognitions can get in the way of seeking out, obtaining, and coping successfully with dental care. There are two steps which must be taken before employing cognitive strategies.

First, you must assess the situation so that you can determine the best way to help the patient. Second, you should provide some information to acquaint the patient with the purposes of the procedure and help the patient develop an optimistic attitude about the procedure's success.

When you observe a patient's behavior and there are clues which indicate the patient is fearful or anxious, it is important to encourage the patient to verbalize the cognitions he is engaging in which may be increasing or perpetuating the anxiety/fear. For example:

"Dave, I notice you're very silent just before I give you an injection and your body seems tense."

"Well, I hate to admit it, but it is something I dread."

"I don't know anyone that enjoys injections, Dave. Your feelings are shared by many others. I know some of my patients find that they have worrisome thoughts or images about the injection procedure before and during it. You know, oftentimes our mental pictures or self-talk do affect the feelings of dread or anxiety we experience."

"I know that I certainly think about it!"

"What do you say to yourself about the injection while you are anticipating it? Are there specific things you say to yourself or mental pictures or images."

"Now that you mention it, there are some thoughts that keep repeating in my mind. I keep thinking, 'I hate this—it's gonna really hurt!' "

In this example the clinician shared an observation regarding the patient's behavior with him and also asked directly about his cognitions. The patient may have responded that he had no related cognitions, but in this case he revealed some specific self-talk which is undoubtedly increasing and maintaining his anxiety and fear.

The next task is to educate the patient so that he understands that his own thinking style affects his fear and anxiety. This may be accomplished simply by stating, "What we say to ourselves, the way we interpret the events around us, has a considerable influence on how we behave. Changing or controlling our thoughts, images, and self-talk can result in changed behavior."

In addition, it is important that the patient believes that he can successfully reduce his fear and anxiety or cope with his pain. His expectation of personal mastery influences his coping abilities. A patient may believe that if he does a particular task certain results will be obtained; but he may not believe that he can do the task. An example of this is the patient who believes he can lose weight if he gives up eating candy, although he does not believe he can give up eating candy. Persuading the patient to try the techniques you are about to teach him and to believe that he can do the procedure will increase the chances of success.

Once cognitions have been changed and modified, the way is prepared for the introduction of a strategy for change. In the following pages are several techniques that you may wish to teach to your patients to enable them better to manage their fears, anxiety, and pain.

Thought Stopping. A quick and highly successful way to interrupt worrying and catastrophizing thoughts or images is through **thought stopping**.

All trays, lights, and the like are moved away from the chair. Asking the patient to close his eyes, listen to his breathing, and let his body relax totally as he exhales will help him relax. The patient is asked to think of the fearful statements or images and to raise a finger when so engaged. The clinician then says loudly, "STOP!" If the patient does not appear too nervous, this may be accompanied by a clap of the hands or stamping of the foot to maximize a startled effect. This usually causes the patient to be mildly startled and interrupts the negative cognitions. Next, the clinician asks the patient to repeat the process, this time with the patient saying "STOP!" out loud. The patient is then instructed to say "STOP!" subvocally whenever fear or anxiety-producing cognitions occur.

It is important to keep in mind that the cognitions should be interrupted at their onset. Sometimes having the patient imagine a red stop sign simultaneously with the saying of "STOP!" adds some impact to the process.

An example of this procedure follows.

"I notice, Mr. Smith, that you're holding onto the chair rather tightly today."

"Yes, I am a little tense. Those injections, you know."

"It sounds as if you're worrying about the injection today."

"Yes, that's right. I always feel tense before the injection."

"You know, Mr. Smith, worrisome thoughts result in tenseness and anxiousness which make what we are anticipating more difficult. Would you like to know how I teach my patients to deal with those thoughts?"

"I sure would. I would love to quit worrying so much."

"All right. Can you tell me a particular thought or image which relates to the injection?"

"Well, one thing that keeps coming to my mind is the picture of the needle plunging into my gum and I can actually feel it, I think."

"I see. Well, the technique I am going to teach you has been highly successful for many of my patients and I believe you can master it without difficulty. I am going to ask you to sit back in the chair and relax. Close your eyes and get comfortable. Listen to your breathing, and with every breath you exhale imagine your body is getting more and more relaxed. In a few seconds I will say the word 'go'. As soon as I say 'go' I want you to imagine the needle plunging into your gum as vividly as you can. As soon as you begin to get the image in your mind, signal me by raising your right index finger. Do you understand the instructions? Good. Sit back, relax, and listen to your breathing.''

(Pause for a few moments to give patient chance to relax.)

"Are you ready? Go."

As the patient raises his finger, the clinician shouts "STOP!" and simultaneously stamps his foot.

"Oh!"

"Where are those thoughts now, Mr. Smith?"

"[Laugh] I'm afraid they went right out of my head."

Subsequently, the patient is taken through the exercise once more. This time the procedure is different in that the patient shouts "STOP!" The patient is then instructed to subvocalize the "STOP!" and to practice this procedure during the appointment and at home. This activity should be reinforced at each visit.

Thought Stopping, Positive Thoughts and Images. An additional step may be added to strengthen the efforts to interrupt and control negative cognitions. After the word "STOP!" is subvocalized, a pleasant statement or image is then used to replace the prior worrisome thoughts. Usually the previously outlined thought-stopping process is enough for the patient to attempt at one time. During the next visit, however, adding an image or positive self-statement to the procedure can be helpful.

In the case of utilizing imagery, a pleasant scene or image is identified by the patient with the help of the clinician. The patient is instructed to think of the pleasant image immediately after the interruption of the catastrophizing thoughts. A variation of this technique may be the utilization of a positive self-statement instead of the pleasant image such as "I did that very well," or "I really have this thing under control."

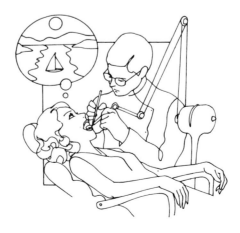

Modeling—With the Patient as the Model. Watching a mental 'movie' of yourself successfully performing a task is an excellent way to learn. Athletes often 'psych' themselves up by mentally picturing themselves doing an athletic feat successfully. In fact, mental practice actually increases our skills for the behavior we actually engage in.

You can capitalize on this method in the operatory. Patients who are anxious or fearful or behave inappropriately can be encouraged to imagine themselves coping effectively with the dental experience. This can be done in the operatory prior to the delivery of dental care or performed by the patient as a homework assignment.

The patient should be encouraged to sit comfortably in a chair, to take two or three deep breaths, and to relax as much as possible. The clinician may suggest that the patient imagine that he is indeed sitting in the dental chair, his teeth are being examined, the clinician is telling him what he wishes to do that day, and the clinician is applying the topical anesthetic. The patient is then asked to imagine the clinician is giving an injection, putting the rubber dam on, and filling the tooth. The patient imagines he is sitting quietly and comfortably during this process and even during times of usual discomfort (which may be different for each patient and should be specified) the patient remains composed and in control of himself. The clinician finishes his task and compliments the patient on his excellent behavior. The patient imagines that he feels good about himself.

The clinician may, in addition, take the patient through a practice session and give a homework assignment.

"To help you feel less anxious about your dental appointments, I would like to give you a home assignment. Would you be willing to spend 15 minutes each day for the three days prior to each appointment preparing for it?"

"If it will help, I will."

"Good. Notice how you feel in the chair and the look, the smell, the sounds around you. [Operates handpiece briefly.] For five minutes, three times a day for the three days prior to your next appointment, I would like you to imagine yourself in the chair here in the operatory. In the 'movie' you mentally play for yourself, imagine you are coming into the room and taking your place in the chair, mentally going through the whole sequence of having your tooth filled. All during this process you notice that you are calm and relaxed. Toward the end of your imaginary appointment, compliment yourself on how competently you handled the entire session. Make it as lifelike as you can and always imagine yourself coping effectively, acknowledging how well you are doing. If you will do that faithfully, I believe you will be pleased at how much better you feel during your appointments."

Written instructions, such as the Rehearsal Card shown here, given to the patient to take home may be helpful as a guide and/or reminder.

Rehearsal Card

Your next appointment is on January 12. On January 9, 10, and 11 you are to spend five minutes, three times a day (15 minutes total) mentally rehearsing your appointment. During the mental rehearsal you are to imagine you are calm and relaxed. Please compliment yourself whenever you do something well in your mental exercise.

Please observe the following steps.

1. Get comfortable in a chair or stretch out on a bed or the floor.
2. Provide for your own privacy so you will not be interrupted.
3. Play the scene as it was rehearsed in the dental office adding any realistic details you like.
4. Emphasize your calmness and competence.
5. Compliment yourself for being such an excellent patient.

Coping Through the Help of Self-Talk. Frequently stress is situational. Patients may not feel stressed during the whole dental appointment, but only at certain times, perhaps during certain procedures. For some, it may be when they first enter the operatory and perceive the sights and smells. For others it may be during the injection process, the placement of the rubber dam, or perhaps only during the time the high speed drill is used.

It is important to pinpoint whether the stress is experienced during the entire appointment or related only to a specific time or procedure. Even if the stress is present during the entire appointment, it is still helpful to encourage the patient to view anxiety or pain as a series of phases rather than one large trauma. In this way the problem is more manageable and the clinician can teach the patient skills in coping with one aspect during one appointment and another at the next.

Teaching the patient self-talk that will help reduce anxiety or response to pain is a technique which can be utilized in a variety of ways in the operatory. An example is presented below.

Billy Osgood is a 9-year-old who does well throughout the restorative appointment except when the rubber dam is put in place. During this procedure he wiggles and fusses. The first task would be to specify whether

Anxiety, Fear, Phobias, and Pain

the rubber dam or the clamp causes the stress, or if it is both. In Billy's case, it is both and the clinician has decided to teach Billy to cope with the dam first. He will teach Billy three steps in doing this—all involving the use of self-talk.

Phase 1 Preparing for stress
Phase 2 Confronting and handling stress
Phase 3 Reinforcing self-statements

The process might go somewhat like this:

"Billy, I see you're wiggling now that it's time to put on the rubber dam. Remember, I told you last week I would teach you how to get on top of those feelings about the dam? It will be a couple of minutes until I put it in place. [Phase 1] Until then, I want you to practice saying to yourself, 'Don't worry, worry won't help' or 'I'll just think about what I will do instead of getting nervous.' Here is my watch; practice your self-talk and tell me when two minutes are up and it is time to put the dam on."

(One minute passes.) "How are you doing, Billy? What are you saying to yourself?"

"I'm saying, 'Don't worry, it's gonna be O.K. No sweat!' "

"Good, Billy, keep it up."

(Another minute passes.) "It's time."

"Fine, Billy, now here is a rubber dam for you to play with. It really stretches, doesn't it. While I am putting this dam on, I want you to say something like, [Phase 2] 'Relax, I can handle this. If I feel nervous I'll just breathe deeply and count to five.' Will you say that for me out loud, Billy? [Billy repeats.] Good, that's the stuff. You're going to do fine. If you do feel nervous, go ahead and count to five. You know, Billy, it's sort of like that old story about The Little Engine That Could. Do you remember that story? The engine kept telling himself, 'I know I can,' and he did what he set out to do. O.K., you start talking to yourself and I'll put the dam on."

(The clinician finishes and Billy does better this time.)

[Phase 3] "You did it, Billy. Really fine. I want you to say to yourself, 'I really did good. I can do it.' "

Some suggestions for self-statements to use during the three phases are listed below. These were largely developed and described in 1974 by Donald Meichenbaum, a major figure in behavioral research.

Phase 1: Preparing for stress

"You can plan a way to deal with it."
"I won't worry—that doesn't help anything."
"Just think about what you can do about it, that's better than getting anxious."

Special Management Considerations

Phase 2: Coping with and handling stress

"Psych yourself up—you can meet this challenge."
"One step at a time—you can handle this situation."
"I know I can do it, just take a deep breath."
"It will be over soon, I'm doing fine."

Phase 3: Reinforcing self-statements

"It worked—I did it!"
"I'm getting better every time."
"I did really well. My self-talk is working."

Summary. These techniques are provided as a sampling of some of the cognitive strategies to reduce and control fear, anxiety, and pain. Some will be more suitable than others for your patients. Their use may seem cumbersome for the first few trials but will become smoother as you gain confidence and skill. Assessment of the patient's problem should help determine which techniques would be most beneficial.

While change can occur quickly, most often it is a gradual process. The practitioner utilizing these techniques should not anticipate immediate results. Some patients have severe problems and the practitioner would be wise to consider referral to a professional who is skilled in helping patients overcome such problems.

Presentation Is Important

We have previously discussed approaches designed to help you change patient home care behavior, and in this chapter we have offered specific techniques which can be used to help the patient cope with anxiety, fear, and pain in the operatory. *The success of these approaches as well as the technical procedures you perform is significantly influenced by your presentation to patients, and by your belief or confidence in those procedures.* This phenomenon is called the **self-fulfilling prophecy** or **expectation effect.**

This effect has been well documented across a number of disciplines. The use of harmless but inert placebo medicines has long been a common medical practice. The effectiveness of placebo drugs is not so surprising, even to the man on the street, as the common term 'sugar pills' illustrates. A striking example of the practitioner's role in making a placebo work can be seen in an experiment in which patients with bleeding ulcers were divided into two groups. Members of the first group were informed by the practitioner that the new drug they were to take would undoubtedly produce relief. The second group was told by nurses that a new, experimental drug would be administered, but that little was known about its effects. Seventy percent of the patients in the first group received significant relief from their ulcers; only 25% of the second group perceived a similar benefit. Both groups received the same placebo drug. The authority and confidence of the practitioner serve as cues to patients that activate their own healing process. Practitioners often discover that technical competence is not enough—it is the patient's belief in the beneficiality of the procedure which is the critical factor in determining the success of the treatment.

In reviewing studies concerned with fear reduction, it has been found that cues, or expectancy factors, are important influences when the placebo produces the same degree of expectation for therapeutic gain as does the 'active' treatment. Similarly, self-fulfilling prophecies or expectations about how we expect others to behave have a significant influence on patient behavior that goes beyond the actual treatment we are providing.

If you expect that the patient will respond positively to your attempt to help him cope with his fear, it may itself be all that is needed. If a person reports that he is afraid and cues are given which grant him 'permission' to be afraid, he will tend to be more fearful than if the expectation is that he will cope adequately. For example, psychiatric experience in the United States Army seems to suggest that the more clearly a psychiatric casualty is treated as such, the less likely it is that he can return to duty.

It is important to note that we are not advocating 'salesmanship' or other forms of 'hype'. Such approaches only leave the patient feeling that you may be trying to put something over on him. What we are saying is that your own self-confidence, voice tone, expectations, sincerity, and all those other unmeasurable qualities which play such a large part in human interactions will influence how the patient feels about dental care, you, and the work that you perform. Technical competence simply is not enough.

Appendix A

Review of the Behavior Change Process

First Session: Steps 1 and 2

Tasks

1. Determine ownership of the problem.
2. If change is desired, determine if the problem is a skill or management deficiency by observing the patient. Could he do it if his life depended on it? If "No," instruct before proceeding.
3. Discuss the importance of finding out when and where the behavior is occurring and not occurring. Arrange for the patient to collect baseline data. A contract may be helpful in making the agreement.

The first step consists of identifying a problem that the patient desires to work on and defining, as specifically as possible, the problem and its probable cause. In other words, what and why. Here we determine if the problem is a skill or a management deficiency. Could the patient brush or floss properly if he had to do it?

The second step is pinpointing—identifying when and where the behavior occurs or does not occur. Prior to attempting to initiate any change, we must find out specific instances of when and where the behavior is occurring and not occurring. For example, a patient who is in college may or may not be aware that he almost never brushes his teeth on weekends or when he has an early morning class. Information on when and where is usually obtained when baseline data are collected and reviewed by the patient and health professional.

Second Session: Steps 3 and 4 (about two weeks later)

Tasks

1. Review baseline data with patient.
2. Set overall goals and realistic and specific intermediate objectives.
3. Plan a strong intervention that uses a number of strategies.
4. Include all relevant information in a contract. Have patient sign it and possibly make it public.

Step 3 consists of examining the baseline data collected by the patient and setting overall goals and realistic intermediate objectives that can be reached.

Instead of requesting patients to brush and floss more often or better, it is more effective to indicate a specific and realistic number of times per week as an intermediate objective.

For example, Ms. Jones, who brushes twice a week, may be successful in increasing her brushing to four times a week. Requesting her to brush and floss every day may be too high a goal to strive for initially and would result in feelings of failure, as there would be no focus on her success in increasing her home care.

Step 4 involves planning and implementing an intervention method. This phase includes deciding what you will actually do to help change the behavior, the results you hope to achieve, and the step-by-step procedure you will follow. To increase your chances of bringing about some positive movement and change, it is wise to bring more than one intervention strategy to bear on the problem if possible. Once the specific goals, objectives, and interventions are agreed upon, a contract is drawn up and signed by both you and the patient.

Third Session: Step 5 (generally two weeks to a month later)

Tasks

1. Review the data collected and charted by the patient.
2. Modify the intervention plan and/or objectives, as needed.
3. Rewrite contract to reflect changes.

Step 5 consists of reviewing and modifying the intervention plan through the remaining phases of the behavior change process. Review data collected and charted by the patient. In doing so, you will be aware of what seems to be going right and what is not working. It is very common for the initial design to have unforeseen weaknesses. More likely than not, some problems will arise. Troubleshoot and modify the intervention plan and/or intermediate objectives or even goals (see chapter 5). Revise or rewrite the contract to reflect these changes.

Fourth Session: Step 6 (generally two weeks to a month later)

Tasks

1. Review the data collected and charted by the patient.
2. Plan for self-maintenance and short- and long-term follow-up.

Step 6 involves terminating the formal change project. Every project has a beginning and an end. The end must be as carefully planned as the beginning to avoid backsliding. Though you have been careful in planning and implementing change in habits and behavior, many people find themselves falling back into old habits and patterns of behavior. Such backsliding should be expected and plans should be made to minimize its effect (see 'Thinning' in chapter 6). Failure to do so may result in the undoing of all change and make renewed efforts at changing behavior more difficult. This step consists of formulating and implementing a self-maintenance plan, and plans for short- and long-term follow-up visits and/or telephone calls.

Appendix B

Guidelines for Choosing Reinforcements

Choosing and constructing a reward system which is actually strong enough to help an individual change his behavior is probably the most important and difficult task in any change project.

The best time to begin attempting to identify reinforcers is when baselines are being taken. If you can determine the antecedents and consequences surrounding an event, and alter them in some way, this will greatly increase your chances of success. When choosing a specific reward, it is critical to choose something the individual will gain if he succeeds at changing his behavior. The reward system should not be set up in such a way that the individual merely stands to lose something, or some activity, if he fails to meet his goals. Following these guidelines is a list which can be utilized to help people think about what kinds of things they find reinforcing. One primary advantage is that it can be filled out any time, and then discussed during a clinic visit.

A final caution. When working with a person living in a family situation, it is important to spend some time inquiring about how the other family members feel about the individual's changing his behavior. This is especially critical if another family member is involved in the project, such as when a husband and wife both try to change oral care together, or when another family member is in charge of dispersing the reward. For example, it may be that the other person might like things as they are, such as when a husband doesn't really want his wife to lose weight; or where one might abuse the reward system to needle or punish the individual who is trying to change.

Reinforcement Survey Schedule*

The items in this questionnaire refer to things and experiences that may give joy or other pleasurable feelings. Check each item in the column that describes how much pleasure it gives you nowadays.

---

* Cautela, J.R., and Kastenbaum, R. Reinforcement schedule for use in therapy, training, and research. Psychol. Rep., 20:1115-1130, 1967 — reprinted by permission of authors and publisher.

Section I

	Not at all	A little	A fair amount	Much	Very much
1. Eating					
a. Ice cream	——	——	——	——	——
b. Candy	——	——	——	——	——
c. Fruit	——	——	——	——	——
d. Pastry	——	——	——	——	——
e. Nuts	——	——	——	——	——
f. Cookies	——	——	——	——	——
2. Beverages					
a. Water	——	——	——	——	——
b. Milk	——	——	——	——	——
c. Soft drink	——	——	——	——	——
d. Tea	——	——	——	——	——
e. Coffee	——	——	——	——	——
3. Alcoholic beverages					
a. Beer	——	——	——	——	——
b. Wine	——	——	——	——	——
c. Hard liquor	——	——	——	——	——
4. Beautiful women	——	——	——	——	——
5. Handsome men	——	——	——	——	——
6. Solving problems					
a. Crossword puzzles	——	——	——	——	——
b. Mathematical problems	——	——	——	——	——
c. Figuring out how something works	——	——	——	——	——
7. Listening to music					
a. Classical	——	——	——	——	——
b. Country & western	——	——	——	——	——
c. Jazz	——	——	——	——	——
d. Show tunes	——	——	——	——	——
e. Rhythm & blues	——	——	——	——	——
f. Rock & roll	——	——	——	——	——
g. Folk	——	——	——	——	——
h. Popular	——	——	——	——	——
8. Nude women	——	——	——	——	——
9. Nude men	——	——	——	——	——
10. Animals					
a. Dogs	——	——	——	——	——
b. Cats	——	——	——	——	——
c. Horses	——	——	——	——	——
d. Birds	——	——	——	——	——

Section II

	Not at all	A little	A fair amount	Much	Very much
11. Watching sports					
a. Football	____	____	____	____	____
b. Baseball	____	____	____	____	____
c. Basketball	____	____	____	____	____
d. Track	____	____	____	____	____
e. Golf	____	____	____	____	____
f. Swimming	____	____	____	____	____
g. Running	____	____	____	____	____
h. Tennis	____	____	____	____	____
i. Pool	____	____	____	____	____
j. Other	____	____	____	____	____
12. Reading					
a. Adventure	____	____	____	____	____
b. Mystery	____	____	____	____	____
c. Famous people	____	____	____	____	____
d. Poetry	____	____	____	____	____
e. Travel	____	____	____	____	____
f. True confessions	____	____	____	____	____
g. Politics & history	____	____	____	____	____
h. How to do it	____	____	____	____	____
i. Humor	____	____	____	____	____
j. Comic books	____	____	____	____	____
k. Love stories	____	____	____	____	____
l. Spiritual	____	____	____	____	____
m. Sexy	____	____	____	____	____
n. Sports	____	____	____	____	____
o. Medicine	____	____	____	____	____
p. Science	____	____	____	____	____
q. Newspapers	____	____	____	____	____
13. Looking at interesting buildings	____	____	____	____	____
14. Looking at beautiful scenery	____	____	____	____	____
15. TV, movies, or radio	____	____	____	____	____
16. Like to sing	____	____	____	____	____
a. Alone	____	____	____	____	____
b. With others	____	____	____	____	____

	Not at all	A little	A fair amount	Much	Very much
17. Like to dance					
a. Ballroom	___	___	___	___	___
b. Discotheque	___	___	___	___	___
c. Ballet or interpretive	___	___	___	___	___
d. Square dancing	___	___	___	___	___
e. Folk dancing	___	___	___	___	___
18. Performing on a musical instrument	___	___	___	___	___
19. Playing sports					
a. Football	___	___	___	___	___
b. Baseball	___	___	___	___	___
c. Basketball	___	___	___	___	___
d. Track & field	___	___	___	___	___
e. Golf	___	___	___	___	___
f. Swimming	___	___	___	___	___
g. Running	___	___	___	___	___
h. Tennis	___	___	___	___	___
i. Pool	___	___	___	___	___
j. Boxing	___	___	___	___	___
k. Judo or karate	___	___	___	___	___
l. Fishing	___	___	___	___	___
m. Skin diving	___	___	___	___	___
n. Auto or cycle racing	___	___	___	___	___
o. Hunting	___	___	___	___	___
p. Skiing	___	___	___	___	___
20. Shopping					
a. Clothes	___	___	___	___	___
b. Furniture	___	___	___	___	___
c. Auto parts/supply	___	___	___	___	___
d. Appliances	___	___	___	___	___
e. Food	___	___	___	___	___
f. New car	___	___	___	___	___
g. New place to live	___	___	___	___	___
h. Sports equipment	___	___	___	___	___
21. Gardening	___	___	___	___	___
22. Playing cards	___	___	___	___	___

	Not at all	A little	A fair amount	Much	Very much
23. Hiking or walking	___	___	___	___	___
24. Completing a difficult job	___	___	___	___	___
25. Camping	___	___	___	___	___
26. Sleeping	___	___	___	___	___
27. Taking a bath	___	___	___	___	___
28. Taking a shower	___	___	___	___	___
29. Being right	___	___	___	___	___
a. Guessing what somebody is going to do	___	___	___	___	___
b. In an argument	___	___	___	___	___
c. About your work	___	___	___	___	___
d. On a bet	___	___	___	___	___
30. Being praised	___	___	___	___	___
a. About your appearance	___	___	___	___	___
b. About your work	___	___	___	___	___
c. About your hobbies	___	___	___	___	___
d. About your physical strength	___	___	___	___	___
e. About your athletic ability	___	___	___	___	___
f. About your mind	___	___	___	___	___
g. About your personality	___	___	___	___	___
h. About your moral strength	___	___	___	___	___
i. About your understanding of others	___	___	___	___	___
31. Having people seek you out for company	___	___	___	___	___
32. Flirting	___	___	___	___	___
33. Having somebody flirt with you	___	___	___	___	___
34. Talking with people who like you	___	___	___	___	___
35. Making somebody happy	___	___	___	___	___
36. Babies	___	___	___	___	___
37. Children	___	___	___	___	___
38. Old women	___	___	___	___	___
39. Old men	___	___	___	___	___
40. Having people ask your advice	___	___	___	___	___
41. Watching other people	___	___	___	___	___
42. Somebody smiling at you	___	___	___	___	___

	Not at all	A little	A fair amount	Much	Very much
43. Making love	——	——	——	——	——
44. Happy people	——	——	——	——	——
45. Being close to an attractive woman	——	——	——	——	——
46. Being close to an attractive man	——	——	——	——	——
47. Talking about the opposite sex	——	——	——	——	——
48. Talking to friends	——	——	——	——	——
49. Being perfect	——	——	——	——	——
50. Winning a bet	——	——	——	——	——
51. Being in church or temple	——	——	——	——	——
52. Saying prayers	——	——	——	——	——
53. Having somebody pray for you	——	——	——	——	——
54. Peace and quiet	——	——	——	——	——

Section III

Situations I Would Like to Be in

How much would you enjoy being in each of the following situations?

1. You have just completed a difficult job. Your superior comes by and praises you highly for a job well done. He also makes it clear that such good work is going to be rewarded very soon.

   not at all ☐   a little ☐   a fair amount ☐   much ☐   very much ☐

2. You are at a lively party. Somebody walks across the room to you, smiles in a friendly way, and says, "I'm glad to meet you. I've heard so many good things about you. Do you have a moment to talk?"

   not at all ☐   a little ☐   a fair amount ☐   much ☐   very much ☐

3. You have just led your team to victory. An old friend comes over and says, "You played a terrific game. Let me treat you to dinner and drinks."

   not at all ☐   a little ☐   a fair amount ☐   much ☐   very much ☐

References

Introduction

Davis, M.S. Variations in patients' compliance with doctors' orders: Analyses of congruence between survey responses and results of empirical investigations. J. Med. Educ. 41:1037-1048, 1966.

Sackett, D.L., and Haynes, R.B. Compliance with Therapeutic Regimens. Baltimore: Johns Hopkins Press, 1976.

Chapter One

Cooper, K.H. The New Aerobics. New York: Bantam Books, 1970.

Mager, R.F. Analyzing Performance Problems. Belmont, California: Fearon Publishers, 1970.

Chapter Four

Bandura, A. Principles of Behavior Modification. New York: Holt, Rinehart and Winston, 1969.

Hall, V.R., et al. Use of self-imposed contingencies to reduce the frequency of smoking behavior. Paper presented at the Association for the Advancement of Behavior Therapy, Washington, D.C., September 1971.

Levitas, T.C. HOME—hand over mouth exercise. J. Dentistry Child. 41:178-182, 1974.

Nolan, J.D. Self-control procedures in the modification of smoking behavior. J. Consulting Clin. Psychol. 32:92-93, 1968.

Nurenberger, S.I., and Zimmerman, J. Applied analyses of human behavior: An alternative to conventional motivational influences and unconscious determination in therapeutic programming. Behavior Ther. 1:59-69, 1970.

Premack, D. Reinforcement theory. In David Levine (Ed.), Nebraska Symposium on Motivation. Lincoln, Nebraska: University of Nebraska Press, pp. 123-188, 1965.

Chapter Seven

Anderson, R., and Anderson, O.W. A Decade of Health Services. Chicago: University of Chicago Press, 1967.

Bhaskar, S.N. Oral lesions in the aged population. Geriatrics 23:137-139, 1968.

Fishman, N., and Bikofsky, C.G. (Eds.). Proceedings of the Conference on Dentistry and the Geriatric Patient. Boston: Harvard School of Dental Medicine, 1972.

Forgione, A., and Clark, E. Comments on an empirical study of the cause of dental fears. J. Dental Res. 53:496, 1974.

Hoyer, W.J., Mishara, B.L., and Riebel, R.G. Problem behaviors as operants. Gerontologist 15:452-456, 1975.

Kastenbaum, R. Perspectives on the development and modification of behavior in the aged. Gerontologist 8:280-283, 1968.

Kleinknecht, R.A., Klepac, R.K., and Alexander, L.D. Origins and characteristics of fear of dentistry. J. Am. Dental Assoc. 86:842-848, 1973.

Lautch, H. Dental phobia. Br. J. Psychiatry 119:151-158, 1971.

Libb, J.W., and Clements, C.B. Token reinforcement in an exercise program for hospitalized geriatric patients. Perceptual and Motor Skills 28:957-958, 1969.

Meichenbaum, D. Cognitive—Behavior Modification. New York: Plenum Press, 1977.

Shoben, E.J., and Borland, L. An empirical study of the etiology of dental fears. J. Clin. Psychol. 10:171-174, 1954.

Siefert, I., Langer, A., and Michmann, J. Evaluation of psychological factors in geriatric denture patients. J. Prosthet. Dentistry 19:516-523, 1972.

Szasz, T., and Hollender, M.H. A contribution to the philosophy of medicine. Arch. Intern. Med. 97:585-592, 1956.

Wright, G.Z. (Ed.). Behavior Management in Dentistry for Children. Philadelphia: W.B. Saunders, 1975.

Wright, G.Z., Alpern, G.D., and Leake, J.L. The modifiability of maternal anxiety as it relates to children's cooperative dental behavior. J. Dentistry Child. 40:265-271, 1973.

Wurster, C., Weinstein, P., and Domoto, P. Identifying functional and dysfunctional patterns of communication in child management. Paper presented to the International Association for Dental Research, Washington, D.C., March 1978.

Chapter Eight

Addelston, H.K. Child patient training. Fort. Rev. Chicago Dent. Soc. 38:7-9, 27-29, 1959.

Crockett, B. Dental survey: Southeastern State College. J. Okla. Dental Assoc. 55:25, 1965.

Friedson, E., and Feldman, J.J. The public looks at dental care. J. Am. Dental Assoc. 53:83-87, 1958.

Holmes, T.H., and Rahe, R.H. The social readjustment rating scale. J. Psychosomatic Res. 11:213, 1967.

Horan, J.J., and Dellinger, J.K. "In vivo" emotive imagery and experimental test. Percept. Mot. Skills. 39:359-362, 1974.

Kleinknecht, R.A., and Bernstein, D. Attitudes and expectations in relation to fear of dentistry. Paper presented to the International Association for Dental Research, Miami, Florida, March 1976.

Kleinknecht, R.A., Klepac, R.K., and Alexander, L.D. Origins and characteristics of fear of dentistry. J. Am. Dental Assoc. 86:842-848, 1973.

Lautch, H. Dental phobia. Br. J. Psychiatry 119:151-158, 1971.

Meichenbaum, D. Self-instructional methods. In Kanter, F.H., and Goldstein, A.P. (Eds.), Helping People Change: A Textbook of Methods. New York: Pergamon Press, 1975.

Papermaster, A.A. A psychological study of the dental patient. Northwest Dentistry 59:149-154, 1971.

Shoben, E.J., and Borland, L. An empirical study of the etiology of dental fears. J. Clin. Psychol. 10:171-174, 1954.

Annotated Bibliography

We would like to suggest various books and articles for interested readers who want more information than we can provide in our small volume. Rather than refer you to journals and monographs that are difficult to obtain, we have cited readily available books and journals. They all offer informative and enjoyable reading.

Behavior Management Skills

The increasing popularity of behavior modification has stimulated the publication of a large number of general training manuals and primers. Behavioral training texts have also appeared for specific topic areas such as child management in the classroom, weight control, interpersonal change, writing behavioral contracts, and self change. These books are written for a lay audience and are relatively free of jargon.

Fordyce, Wilbert E. Behavioral Methods for Chronic Pain and Illness. St. Louis: C. V. Mosby, 1976, 236 pp.

Although not written with dental personnel in mind, this book contains concepts and procedures that are extremely valuable. The text is divided into three sections: (1) Contemporary theories of pain, the effect of learning on pain behavior, the acquisition of pain, and techniques of behavioral analysis and change; (2) Applying behavioral techniques previously discussed to the assessment of chronic pain patients; and (3) Management procedures for such patients.

Mager, Robert F., and Pipe, Peter. Analyzing Performance Problems. Belmont, California: Fearon Publishers, 1970, 109 pp.

This easy-to-read little soft-covered book is definitely a gem and should be required reading for all health professionals and educators. The authors provide the reader with a frame of reference in which to diagnose human performance problems—especially when someone is not doing what he should be doing. "Key Issues" and "Questions to Ask" are clearly outlined. The flow-charts and "Quick Reference Checklist" alone are worth the modest price of this book.

Schmidt, Jurg A. Help Yourself. Champaign, Illinois: Research Press, 1976, 119 pp.

This small, jargon-free, soft-covered book is an attempt to popularize basic information about behavior change to readers who want to sort out some of their problems and to change without professional help. The author specifies a number of general strategies and provides helpful examples. Chapter headings are informative—they include: "Becoming a self-watcher," "What triggers you to act," "Increasing motivation with payoffs," and "Self-contracting."

Stuart, Richard B., and Davis, Barbara. Slim Chance in a Fat World. Champaign, Illinois: Research Press, 1972, 245 pp.

The authors of this manual have put together what we believe to be the most comprehensive behavioral weight-loss program. This paperback guide to sustained weight reduction includes three key elements: behavioral control of eating, nutrition management, and management of exercise. The behavioral control chapters present strategy after strategy that can be used to great advantage. Though the book is well documented and academically oriented, it may be appropriate reading for the general public.

Van Zoost, Brenda (Ed.). Psychological Readings for the Dental Profession. Chicago: Nelson Hill, 1975, 176 pp.

This volume of psychologically-oriented papers published in dental journals is divided into three sections: (1) Communication and management of dental patients (6 papers); (2) Management of dental patient anxiety (6 papers); and (3) Motivation of dental patients (5 papers). The book is heavily oriented toward the young patient and toward the application of behavioristic approaches to dentistry.

Watson, David L., and Tharp, Roland G. Self-Directed Behavior. Monterey, California: Brooks/Cole Publishing Company, 1977, 238 pp.

This hard-covered textbook is now in its second edition and is even more readable and useful than the first edition. Though the book attempts to guide the novice, step-by-step, through a self-change program, it is also useful for helping others work through their own program of change. The text is oriented toward a college-level student audience and is relatively complete. The authors explain basic psychological principles, give references for relevant research, and specify how and when to use a variety of clinical behavior change techniques. Separate chapters are devoted to observing and recording data, antecedents, consequences, and developing new behaviors (including relaxation, troubleshooting, and termination).

Communication Skills

There are many useful books about communicating that warrant review. A few that focus on communicating with children will be cited in the Child Management Skills section of this bibliography. Though a number of books are written to guide health professionals, few are as well done as Endow and Swisher's medically-oriented volume, Interviewing and Patient Care (1972). On the other hand, there is only one book that specifically addresses communication in dental settings.

Froelich, Robert E., Bishop, F. Marian, and Dworkin, Samuel F. Communication in the Dental Office. St. Louis: C.V. Mosby Company, 1976, 151 pp.

After preliminary notes about choosing the dental office, initial patient contact, and office setting, the authors provide detailed discussion of how to conduct the various phases of a patient interview. A specific chapter is devoted to nonverbal communication. Many exercises are included in each chapter, and an entire section covers practice interviews and role playing material.

Child Management Skills

Many useful books have been written about how to communicate with and manage children. Gordon's Parent Effectiveness Training (1972) and Haim Ginott's Between Parent and Child (1969) are useful books for dental personnel as well as parents. Many behaviorally oriented books have been written on how to toilet train children, how to manage children in the classroom and in the home, and how to train the mentally retarded. Useful articles often appear in the Journal of Dentistry for Children, published by the American Society of Dentistry for Children. There is even a section of the journal entitled "Behavior." However, at present there is only one text that focuses on the management of child behavior in the dental setting.

Wright, Gerald Z. (Ed). Behavior Management in Dentistry for Children. Philadelphia: W. B. Saunders, 1975, 266 pp.

This hard-covered text provides a scholarly overview of many child management procedures. Current research is integrated with the experience of the 18 contributors. Part 1 provides a thorough but academic introduction to theories of developmental and child psychology. Part 2, which is most valuable, covers pharmacological and nonpharmacological techniques of child management. In addition, in this section there are chapters which cover the use of hypnosis and special considerations for the handicapped and hospitalized. Part 3 presents an approach to training office personnel, the use of group and family therapy, and a thought-provoking chapter on office design.

Index

and dealing with parents, 84-85;
 parental questionnaire, 79-80;
 pre-appointment letter, 84, 100
desensitizing, 102
and hand-over-mouth procedure, 48
interaction model for dentist-child
 relationship, 82-84
misbehavior of, 52, 78; and punishment,
 48; and reinforcement, 65
and office atmosphere, 81
and Premack principle, 40
scheduling, 81, 102-103
and tell-show-do technique, 103
treatment goals for, 77
variables influencing behavior, 80-81
Communication
 with children, 48, 78-79, 82-85
 with elderly patients, 88-90
 with fearful patients, 100-101, 104
 with parents, 84-85
Consequences
 defined, 34-36
 identification of, 36-37
 punishment as, 47
 uses of, to change behavior, 38-39
 see also Reinforcement and reinforcers
Contracts, 18-19, 43, 44, 45, 50
 examples of, 21-22, 61
Cueing, see Prompting
Cues, see Antecedents

Dentures, 55, 87, 89
Desensitizing, 102-103

Elderly patients
 and behavior change techniques,
 88-90
 communication with, 85, 88-90
 dental needs of, 86-87
 and dentures, 87, 89
 guidelines for treatment of 77, 85-86,
 88-90
Ethics, 7-8, 46-47
Extinction, 52-53, 65

Fading, 33
Fear, see Anxiety and fear
Feedback, 33, 39, 42-43, 59
Flossing
 contracts for, 21, 22, 61
 counting techniques for, 13

improvement chart for, 57, 59
and Premack principle, 39
and prompting, 32
setting goals for, 25
and shaping, 55, 56
teaching elderly patients, 90

Goal-setting, 15, 20, 25-27
 and baseline counts, 10
 intermediate objectives, 25-26; during
 intervention phase, 54
Grandma's law, see Premack principle

Hand-over-mouth technique, 48, 49
Hands-on prompting, 32
Headgear compliance
 setting goals for, 10, 26
 and shaping, 55

Identifying and defining problems, xv, 3-5
 practice projects, 6-7
Insight, x, 6
Intermediate objectives, see Goal-setting;
 Shaping
Intervention, xvi, 20
 designing a plan, 54-61
 monitoring and modifying, 63-66
 punishment as, 49
 techniques to establish new behavior
 patterns, 30-34; to increase existing
 behavior, 34-47; to decrease
 inappropriate behavior, 47-54

Management deficiencies; 4-5, 93
 and increasing existing behavior,
 34-47
 and decreasing undesirable behavior,
 47-54
 and anxiety and fears, 93
 see also Anxiety and fear
Modeling
 and learning new behavior, 31-32, 33
 and reducing anxiety, 32, 104-105,
 112-113
Monitoring, xvi, 63-66
 self-monitoring, 70
Motivating patients, x, xii-xiv

Nailbiting
  counting techniques for, 14
  and timing of reinforcement, 64
  setting objectives, 25
  and shaping, 56
  techniques to eliminate, 49, 52

Overeating, 50-51, 64, 65
  see also Snacking; Weight loss
Ownership of problems, xiii-xiv, 12

Pain, 95, 97-98, 102
Performance discrepancy, 3-4
Phobias, 95
  see also Anxiety and fear
Pinpointing, *see* Baseline data
Premack principle, 39-40, 71
Preventive dentistry
  and behavior modification, ix-xi
Prompting, 32, 52
Punishment, 47-48
  and oral health habits, 49-50

Reinforcement and reinforcers
  and baseline counting, 47, 63
  and cheating, 59
  continuous, 45
  and extinction, 52-53
  feedback, 42-43
  and frequency of behavior, 65-66
  guidelines for choosing, 40-44, 45, 64,
    120
  immediate, 64
  of incompatible behavior, 53-54
  and punishment, 47
  and shaping, 54-57
  social reinforcement, 42-44
  thinning, 69
  timing of, 64
  tokens, 44
  see also Feedback; Premack principle

Self-talk
  and anxiety, 107-109
  thought-stopping techniques, 110-111
  use of, in controlling anxiety, 113-115
Shaping, 54-59
Skill deficiencies, 4-5
  and pinpointing, 12

remediating by modeling, 31-32; by
    prompting, 32
Smoking
  charting, 57
  and shaping, 56- 57
  techniques to reduce, 50-51, 51-52, 53
  and timing of reinforcement, 64
Snacking, 51-52, 53, 54
  see also Overeating; Weight loss
Stimulus control, 51-52
Structuring of time, 38, 83, 104-105

Tell-show-do technique, 103- 104
Termination, xvi, 69-72
  follow-up, 70-72
  self-monitoring, 70
Thinning, 69
Thumbsucking
  counting techniques for, 14
  techniques for reducing, 53
Tokens, 44
Toubleshooting, 63-66

Weight loss
  monitoring, 71
  setting objectives for, 25
  shaping, 25